THE
Body Sense Natural Diet

THE Body Sense Natural Diet

Six Weeks to a Slimmer, Healthier You

LORNA R. VANDERHAEGHE, B.SC.

WILEY

John Wiley & Sons Canada, Ltd.

Library and Archives Canada Cataloguing in Publication

Vanderhaeghe, Lorna R.
    The body sense natural diet : six weeks to a slimmer,
    healthier you / Lorna Vanderhaeghe. — 1st ed.

Includes index.

ISBN 0-470-83366-1

1. Reducing diets.	I. Title.	
RM222.2.V33 2004	613.2'5	C2004-906086-4

Production Credits:

Cover design: Interrobang Graphic Design Inc.
Interior text design: Adrian So R.G.D.
Front cover photo: Getty Images
Printer: Tri-Graphic Printing Ltd.

John Wiley & Sons Canada, Ltd
6045 Freemount Blvd
Mississauga, Ontario
L5R 4J3

Printed in Canada
10 9 8 7 6 5 4 3 2 1

Contents

Acknowledgements   vii

Introduction   1

Chapter 1   Deadly Weight   5

Chapter 2   Tell Me How Right Now   25

Chapter 3   Emotional Eating   81

Chapter 4   Your Hormones and Weight Gain   99

Chapter 5   Digestive Health   129

Chapter 6   Weight-Loss Supplements   153

Chapter 7   Fast, Fun Fitness   177

Chapter 8   Conquering Cellulite   203

Chapter 9   Natural Treatment for Diabetes   223

Appendix   Recommended Products and Resources   249

Index   253

Acknowledgements

There are always special people who help get a book published. I would like to acknowledge a few of them. First, thank you to Michael Murray, N.D. for your kindness and support since I have joined the Natural Factor's science team.

Deane Parkes, my longtime friend and kindred spirit, you continually provide me with everything I need to be successful. John Morgenthaler, thank you for being a fabulous mentor and loving friend. To the editors at Wiley, your expertise is invaluable.

To my children, Crystal, Kevin, Kyle and Caitlyn, who endured and supported me during the research and writing of this book—I am blessed to have each of you.

Special thanks to the pioneers, physicians and scientists in the fields of obesity and endocrinology: without you, this book would not exist.

For all those persons who have been struggling with weight gain, this book is dedicated to you.

Introduction

"I never worry about diets. The only carrots that interest
me are the number you get in a diamond."
— Mae West —

Mae West may have been on to something when it comes to diets. The sad fact is that most diets don't work because they fail to look at the underlying cause of weight gain and only focus on caloric intake, carbohydrate or protein consumption, and increased exercise. All these factors are important, but all you dieters who have run thousands of miles on the treadmill and eaten buckets of carrot sticks must know by now that there is more to weight loss than just eating low-calorie foods, exercising, and using a lot of willpower.

During the research for *The Body Sense Natural Diet*, I read every diet book currently in print and thousands of research papers. Most diet books provide good advice that, if followed long-term, would help you lose some weight. But the sad story is that most dieters gain back one- to two-thirds of the weight they lost by the end of the first year, and almost all the weight will be gained back (and more!) within five years. The question is why. Stress, emotions, aging, and other factors play a role.

Introduction

The key to permanent weight loss is well hidden. It lies in understanding how each component of dieting affects the hormones that stimulate, regulate, and control thousands of functions in your body. Those hormones conspire to make your fat cells bigger, increase your cravings, tell you to eat more, lower your fat-burning rate, and disrupt your blood sugar. None of the diet books I read explain this or integrate the knowledge into their advice, and yet there are mountains of research on the hormones of obesity.

Within the pages of this book you will find the latest scientific breakthroughs in fat loss—including which hormones are conspiring to make you fat. By using foods, nutrients, and other factors, you can correct hormonal imbalances and reset your body's fat-burning furnace, making weight loss much easier.

The Body Sense Natural Diet is a simple guide that takes you through the hormonal maze and unlocks secrets to diet success. You must normalize key hormones to lose weight and keep it off. Once you understand how foods and lifestyle factors affect your hormones and make you fat or thin, you will recognize why other diets don't work.

Why am I sure it's hormones? Think about it. Menopausal women have been telling their doctors for decades that the hormonal change they experience during this time of transition leads to weight gain that is very difficult to shed. Women taking hormone replacement therapy, including estrogen and progestin, also notice large weight gains and are unable to lose that weight. Research has proven that low thyroid slows your metabolic rate and causes you to gain weight and resist weight loss. Carbohydrate cravings are directly linked to the hormone serotonin, your feel-good hormone. When serotonin is low, your body desires sweet, starchy foods to bring serotonin back to desired levels; nothing will stop you from eating the wrong foods as you satisfy your body's need for this hormone. Cortisol, your stress hormone, is directly linked to making fat cells resistant to fat loss.

Poor digestive-tract health is also linked to weight gain. Poor digestion, candida yeast, and bacteria overgrowth cause the secretion of hormones that expand your pants size. Fat cells themselves are hormone factories: the more fat cells you have, and the bigger they are, the more trouble you will have losing weight. The research is clear—hormones are key to losing those unwanted pounds and keeping them off for good.

The Body Sense Natural Diet is about making sense of nutrition and the hormones of obesity. Natural foods are the focus. By eating organic foods whenever they are available, you will be able to avoid the chemicals and added hormones that are contributing to your weight problems. Adopt the easy-to-use and inexpensive techniques you'll find in the book. This diet does not require you to measure and weigh your food; nor do you have to purchase expensive diet foods. You do not have to take time out of your busy day to enjoy lifelong weight management. This book is more than a diet book. You will learn how to prevent and treat diabetes, low thyroid function, and exhausted adrenal glands; banish cellulite; stop yeast infections and constipation; and much more. The exercise program is fun and takes only 10 minutes per day.

This book is for kids, too. Obesity is affecting the self-esteem and health of children. One in four children between the ages of two and five are obese, and Type 2 diabetes is a real threat for children. You must change the diet of your entire family. This book offers a new way of eating—one that your family will embrace. You won't be making two sets of meals; this eating program is all about food that is delicious and healthy.

After researching and writing many health books, I have concluded that until you achieve a healthy weight, few of the nutritional recommendations or supplements for disease conditions will work effectively. Reducing weight is the key to eliminating so many diseases that obesity should be the first condition to be tackled.

Enjoy this book. Envision yourself as a fit, healthy person. Empty your cupboards of all the toxic, hormone-disrupting foods and start eating healthy foods for permanent weight loss and vibrant health. Over the past several years, thousands of men and women have successfully lost weight and kept it off using this natural diet program. You can be one of them. I receive hundreds of e-mails, letters, and phone calls every day from people just like you who want to change their lives. How will you be rewarded by adopting the recommendations in this book? Optimal health, weight loss, and a new zest for life will be your gifts to yourself.

Deadly Weight

North Americans are obsessed with their weight. According to the U.S. Federal Trade Commission more than U.S. $36 billion annually is spent on weight-loss products. Despite this enormous outlay of money, we are more overweight than ever. Every day a new miracle diet product promises to help us lose weight in record time. Advertising headlines scream, "Increase fat loss by 500 percent and lose 10 pounds in one week." While poor nutrition, specifically in the form of high-fat diets, bears most of the blame for the surge in overweight individuals, our expanding girth is associated with many factors. Manufacturers of weight-loss products capitalize on the latest and greatest diet craze, promoting high-protein, low-carbohydrate, herbal miracles, or liquid diets. The fact is that fad products and diets don't work. They lead to binge eating and repeated cycles of weight gain and loss, and are emotionally and physically destructive due to their restrictive nature. In short, they are harmful to your health.

The Body Sense Natural Diet is like no other diet book. We now have the evidence that being overweight has to do with the dozens of hormones our body produces and how the foods we eat, the lifestyle we live, and the types of exercise we perform affect those hormones. Certain hormones tell us we are hungry, let us know when we are full, cause our fat cells to store fat, while other hormones increase our metabolic rate, soothe our emotional needs, and help us lose weight. *The Body Sense Natural Diet* provides the solutions to normalize our disrupted hormones and burn fat faster using food, exercise, and nutritional supplements. You will be shocked to learn that some of the foods you thought were "diet" foods cause hormones in the body to slow your metabolism and cause your fat cells to become resistant to fat loss.

Scientists have recently learned that fat cells act like hormone factories; the more fat cells you have the more hormones are spewed out, furthering weight gain. Hormones in your digestive tract also contribute to your weight problems, especially when they become disrupted due to food choices, bacterial, viral, or parasitic infections, and bowel habits. Certain foods, like refined carbohydrates and sugar, can trigger the secretion of dozens of hormones that tell your brain you are in need of more food, cause cravings for the wrong foods, and promote severe crashes in the hormones controlling your moods, thus creating a vicious cycle of binge eating and weight gain. Toxic hormones created by man are found in common household cleaning agents, cosmetics, foods, and plastics, and more are being stored in your fat cells. These environmental hormones disrupt the way your body's hormones function, create disease, and cause abdominal weight gain. For decades women have been saying their hormones have been the cause of their weight gain; now we know this to be true. If you have tried dozens of diets with limited success it is because those diets did not address the key component to weight management—your hormones.

Long-term studies show that one-third to two-thirds of the weight lost through dieting is regained within one year, and almost all weight is regained within five years. Faced with this fact, are you wondering why you should even bother trying? Fat loss is not about dieting; it is about eating for a long, healthy life. Diets are considered a success only if weight loss is permanent and you have gained energy and vitality in the process. Diets should satisfy all nutritional needs, be delicious, meet individual tastes and habits, minimize hunger, and boost energy. The cornerstone to successful weight loss is enjoying a moderate lifestyle consisting of healthy foods and lots of love, laughter, friends, and family. But with most of us working what feels like twenty-four hours, seven days a week, raising our families and trying to keep our bills paid, eating for optimal health and weight control is the last thing on our priority list. This is where *The Body Sense Natural Diet* shines. The goal of this diet is to help you adopt healthy eating habits forever. By the time you finish the 42-day program, you will have learned which foods cause hormone imbalances and weight gain, deprive you of energy, and increase your susceptibility to disease. And you will discover all the healthy foods that you should be eating, not just to maintain a healthy weight but also to extend your lifespan and increase your vitality. Not just you but your family, too. You know you can't stay on a diet where you are cooking one thing for yourself and something else for your family. *The Body Sense Natural Diet* is so simple, delicious, and healthy that your entire family will enjoy eating it. This is especially important when you look at the fact that your children are suffering the effects of weight gain, too. Obesity and being overweight constitute the second leading cause of preventable death (after smoking), resulting in an estimated 300,000 deaths annually in the U.S., according to the U.S. Surgeon-General's *Call to Action to Prevent and Decrease Overweight and Obesity* report published in 2001. Obesity is the most common nutritional disorder in the industrialized world today. Data from the United States between 1990 and 2000 show a 65 percent increase in obesity and a 25 percent increase in overweight individuals, resulting in 34 percent of the population being overweight and another 27 percent being obese. This means that more than 60 percent of the U.S. population has a weight problem. The picture is much the same in Canada. The Canadian Community Health Survey reported that 48 percent of the Canadian population is overweight and 15 percent is classified as obese. That is one in seven Canadians.

OVERWEIGHT CHILDREN

For children, the statistics are even more alarming. According to the *National Longitudinal Survey of Children and Youth*, more than a third of Canadian children aged two to eleven are overweight, and half of those are obese. More boys than girls were found to be overweight, and preschoolers fared the worst, with one in four children between the ages of two and five being obese. *The Report on America's Children*, prepared by the U.S. National Institutes of Health and the U.S. Census Bureau, contains similar statistics. That is a lot of fat toddlers, and they are not the ones buying the groceries or driving to fast-food restaurants. We must change the way we feed our children. Aside from the health problems associated with being an overweight child, the emotional issues are quite damaging. We know that overweight children are treated differently by teachers and classmates, resulting in lower self-esteem, which further exacerbates the psychological aspects of eating. I know myself that being a chubby kid was torment. No parent wants this for his or her child. This plan works for the whole family.

YOUR PERSONAL STARTING POINT

The first step in your battle with weight is to take a look at how you live now. By understanding your habits, good and bad, you're more likely to succeed in your quest to be a healthier weight.

Factors That Make Us Fat

Take the following quiz to evaluate the factors that are contributing to the challenges with your weight.

Yes/No

___ Do you drink more than 2 cups coffee or other caffeinated beverages daily?

___ Do you eat artificial sweeteners or non-dairy creamers (fake foods)?

___ Do you drink alcohol more than twice per week?

___ Are you taking prescription or over-the-counter medications (including ___ painkillers and anti-inflammatory medications)?

___ If you take thyroid medication, has your doctor had to increase your ___ dosage more than once?

___ Do you sleep at least eight hours per night?

___ Do you eat hydrogenated or partially hydrogenated foods?

___ Do you take birth-control pills or hormone-replacement therapy (estro- ___ gen and/or progestins)?

___ Have you taken antibiotics in the last year?

___ Are you afraid to eat foods containing fat?

___ Do you choose foods that are fat-free over those that are not?

___ Do you crave certain foods (bread, sweets, pasta)?

___ Do you eat at fast-food restaurants?

___ Do you eat processed foods (processed cheese, meat, or frozen dinners)?

___ Do you eat fewer than two servings of protein per day (eggs, milk, fish, ___ beef, chicken, or tofu)?

___ Do you drink fewer than eight glasses of water per day?

____ Are you stressed (too many things to do and not enough time in the day)?

____ Do you skip breakfast?

____ Do you avoid exercising?

____ Do you eat the food left on your children's plates?

____ Are you sad, angry, stressed, or depressed?

____ Do you view food as a necessary evil?

____ Do you have an overweight extended family?

____ Do you cook and eat the way your family has for generations?

If you said yes to more than six of these questions you will love what you are going to learn in future chapters. Here is a preview.

- Taking estrogen replacement therapy causes low thyroid-hormone production and slows your metabolism so it does not burn fat very efficiently
- Taking antibiotics or anti-inflammatory medications disables the hormones in your digestive tract that tell your brain you are full, which can cause you to overeat
- Skipping breakfast lowers your fat-burning rate dramatically
- If you crave sugar and other refined carbohydrates you may be deficient in a hormone called serotonin, which is necessary for happy moods and the control of how much food you eat
- Fake sugars and non-dairy creamers disrupt the work of your liver, which is where all your hormones are processed and packaged

Each question in the quiz is related to how your food choices and lifestyle factors contribute to being overweight or obese. Future chapters will teach you how to understand, optimize and normalize body functions for maximum weight loss.

THE COST OF WEIGHING TOO MUCH

The rise in excess weight and obesity is now recognized by the World Health Organization as a devastating problem with numerous health implications and public health costs. According to the U.S. Surgeon General, the direct and indirect costs of treating obesity in the United States are approximately $117 billion annually. In Canada, the Canadian Medical Association states the figure is $3.2 billion. This epidemic is a time bomb for heart disease,

Type 2 diabetes, cancer, arthritis, sleep apnea, and many other health complications. As our population ages and our waistbands expand, health care costs will skyrocket even further. Although most people lose weight with the goal of fitting into a smaller dress or pant size, being fat has unhealthy consequences because it takes years off our lives, and the emotional, physical, and societal costs are exorbitant. Pharmaceutical companies are pumping billions of dollars into new weight-loss drugs to fight the war against excess fat, while scientists are trying to unlock and manipulate the genes that make us fat, hoping to develop a vaccine that will keep us all thin. However, the secret, as you will discover, is in the pages of this book.

OBESITY DEFINED

So how do you determine your ideal weight, and whether you are overweight or obese? There are many methods, including the relationship between height and weight, waist circumference, waist-to-hip ratio, and body fat skin fold measurements.

Body Mass Index

But the most common method is the body mass index (BMI). Techniques for measuring excess fat have varied over the years. Underwater weighing is still the gold standard for assessing total body fat. In this method, a person is submerged underwater, then lean body mass and the amount of body fat are calculated. The equipment to do this is costly, so in large human studies and clinical practice, body fat is most typically estimated using the BMI. Hundreds of studies have confirmed the body mass index to be one of the most accurate ways to determine when extra pounds translate into health risks.

A healthy BMI is 24 or less. The U.S. Department of Health and Human Services and the World Health Organization have defined being overweight as a BMI of 25–30, and obesity as a BMI greater than 30.

The higher the BMI, the greater the risk of developing health problems; however, one variable the BMI fails to consider is lean body mass (tissue, bone, and muscle), which weighs significantly more than fat. It is possible for a healthy, muscular individual to be classified as obese using the BMI formula. If you are a trained athlete, your weight based on a measured percentage of body fat would be a better indicator of what you should weigh. A normal healthy man should not exceed 15 percent body fat, while the healthy limit for a woman is 15–22 percent.

Body Mass Index (BMI) Table

BMI	19	20	21	22	23	24	25	26	27	28	29	30	31	32	33	34	35
Height							*Weight (in Pounds)*										
4'10"	91	96	100	105	110	115	119	124	129	134	138	143	148	153	158	162	167
4'11"	94	99	104	109	114	119	124	128	133	138	143	148	153	158	163	168	173
5'	97	102	107	112	118	123	128	133	138	143	148	153	158	163	168	174	179
5'1"	100	106	111	116	122	127	132	137	143	148	153	158	164	169	174	180	185
5'2"	104	109	115	120	126	131	136	142	147	153	158	164	169	175	180	186	191
5'3"	107	113	118	124	130	135	141	146	152	158	163	169	175	180	186	191	197
5'4"	110	116	122	128	134	140	145	151	157	163	169	174	180	186	192	197	204
5'5"	114	120	126	132	138	144	150	156	162	168	174	180	186	192	198	204	210
5'6"	118	124	130	136	142	148	155	161	167	173	179	186	192	198	204	210	216
5'7"	121	127	134	140	146	153	159	166	172	178	185	191	198	204	211	217	223
5'8"	125	131	138	144	151	158	164	171	177	184	190	197	203	210	216	223	230
5'9"	128	135	142	149	155	162	169	176	182	189	196	203	209	216	223	230	236
5'10"	132	139	146	153	160	167	174	181	188	195	202	209	216	222	229	236	243
5'11"	136	143	150	157	165	172	179	186	193	200	208	215	222	229	236	243	250
6'	140	147	154	162	169	177	184	191	199	206	213	221	228	235	242	250	258
6'1"	144	151	159	166	174	182	189	197	204	212	219	227	235	242	250	257	265
6'2'	148	155	163	171	179	186	194	202	210	218	225	233	241	249	256	264	272
6'3'	152	160	168	176	184	192	200	208	216	224	232	240	248	256	264	272	279

Source: Evidence Report of Clinical Guidelines on the Identification, Evaluation, and Treatment of Overweight and Obesity in Adults, 1998. NIH/National Heart, Lung, and Blood Institute (NHLBI)

How to Calculate Your BMI

The BMI is calculated by dividing your weight in kilograms by the square of your height in meters—weight (kg)/height squared (m2). However, most North Americans know their measurements in pounds and inches, so I have provided that calculation.

$$BMI = \frac{(\text{Weight in Pounds})}{(\text{height in inches} \times \text{height in inches})} \times 703$$

Let's say you are five foot six inches tall and you weigh 150 pounds. Five feet 6 inches is 66 inches. So you would multiply 66 by 66, which equals 4,356. Next, take your weight in pounds and divide it by your height squared: divide 150 by 4,356, giving you 0.034. Take the answer and multiply it by 703, which gives you 24.2.

Understanding Your BMI

The *Clinical Guidelines on the Identification, Evaluation and Treatment of Overweight and Obesity in Adults* say that a person with a body mass index (BMI) of more than 30 is obese. A person with a BMI of 25 to 30 is considered overweight.

Extremely, lean well-muscled athletes can not use the BMI as a measure of being overweight or obese. It is not accurate for them because muscle weighs far more than fat. People of this body type use skin-fold measurements, waist circumference, or waist-to-hip ratio to determine ideal weight. In any case, if you are more than 100 lbs (45 kg) over your ideal weight, you are considered morbidly obese and at high risk of death from your excess weight.

Ideal Weight to Height Chart for Adults*

Height	Weight (pounds)		Height	Weight (pounds)		Height	Weight (pounds)	
	Women	Men		Women	Men		Women	Men
4' 10"	92-121	—	5' 4"	110-142	114-145	5' 10"	134-169	137-172
4' 11"	95-124	—	5' 5"	114-146	117-149	5' 11"	—	141-177
5' 0"	98-127	—	5' 6"	118-150	121-154	6' 0"	—	145-182
5' 1"	101-130	105-134	5' 7"	122-154	125-159	6' 1"	—	149-187
5' 2"	104-134	108-137	5' 8"	126-159	129-163	6' 2"	—	153-192
5' 3"	107-138	111-141	5' 9"	130-164	133-167	6' 3"	—	157-197

*Height is without shoes; weight is without clothes.

OUR EXPANDING GIRTH

Waist circumference is another method to determine how overweight you are. Measure your waist circumference with a tape measure comfortably around the smallest area below your rib cage and above your belly button. Women with a waist measurement greater than 35 in (89 cm), combined with a high BMI, are considered obese and at high risk for certain diseases, including heart disease, diabetes, and especially breast cancer. For men, a waist circumference greater than 40 in (102 cm) is a risk factor. Total over-all body fat is still considered the determining factor when looking at weight management. Another method is the waist-to-hip ratio, a mathematical formula that has been scientifically defined. To determine your waist-to-hip ratio, measure the widest part of your buttocks. Take your waist measurement and divide it by your hip measurement. For example, if you have a 30-in (76-cm) waist and 37-in (94-cm) hips, your waist-to-hip ratio is 0.81. For both men and women, a waist-to-hip ratio of 1.0 or greater is considered a risk factor for serious health conditions. The optimal waist-to-hip ratio would be 0.80 for women and 0.90 for men.

Classification of Overweight and Obesity by BMI, Waist Circumference, and Associated Disease Risks

	BMI (kg/m2)	Obesity Class	Disease Risk* Relative to Normal Weight and Waist Circumference †	
			Men 102 cm (40 in) or less Women 88 cm (35 in) or less	Men > 102 cm (40 in) Women > 88 cm (35 in)
Underweight	< 18.5	—	—	—
Normal	18.5 – 24.9	—	—	—
Overweight	25.0 – 29.9	—	Increased	High
Obesity	30.0 – 34.9	I	High	Very High
	35.0 – 39.9	II	Very High	Very High
Extreme Obesity	40.0 +	III	Extremely High	Extremely High

* Disease risk for Type 2 diabetes, hypertension, and heart disease.
† Increased waist circumference can also be a marker for increased risk even in people of normal weight.
U.S. National Heart, Lung, and Blood Institute (NHLBI).

I know that if you are reading this book, you don't need BMI, waist circum-ference, or hip-to-waist ratios to tell you that you need to lose some weight. Though that information has real value, what you really want to know is why you are getting fat and how you can lose weight more effectively.

SEVEN FACTORS THAT MAKE US FAT

Old theories about weight loss were based on the calories in, calories out model. Simply put, the theory was that if you ate less food and exercised more, weight loss would occur. Those who exercise daily, eat salad and carrot sticks, drink glass after glass of water, and still don't lose weight can vouch for the fact that weight loss is not that simple. And we all know people who eat whatever they want, never set foot on a treadmill, and don't put on a pound.

Billions of dollars in health care and related costs are spent on obesity. Now, government organizations, universities, and pharmaceutical compa-nies are funding an explosion of research into fat loss. Scientists have shown that a complex interplay of hormonal, biochemical, genetic, physi-cal, and lifestyle factors are causing our battle of the bulge. The seven factors that make us fat are:

1. basal metabolic rate
2. hormones that regulate weight
3. stress
4. food choices
5. lack of exercise
6. liver dysfunction
7. genetics

1. Basal Metabolic Rate

Your basal metabolic rate (BMR) is the rate at which your body burns calo-ries when you are at rest. Many factors affect your metabolic rate, among them thyroid hormones and how much you exercise. When you hear people refer to their slow metabolism, they are really saying that they have a low BMR. Metabolism is the chemical reactions that take place inside our cells to create energy. All the fuel we eat—carbohydrates, fats, essential fats, and proteins—is broken down to produce the energy we need to maintain our body temperature, breathe, move our muscles, and more. A peak operating metabolism can burn up a lot of fuel (food) and create plenty of energy. Conversely, a slow metabolism will store fuel as fat. The process in which stored fat is burned is known as thermogenesis. *The Body Sense Natural Diet* program is designed to rev up your fat-burning furnace to burn fuel more effectively and use up stored fat.

2. Hormones that Regulate Weight

Dozens of hormones determine whether you stay slim or gain weight. A new field of medicine has been developed to learn more about the delicate interplay of hormones and how they affect fat cells. We now know that fat cells manufacture their own hormones, which makes losing weight even more difficult. Following chapters provide new insight into how to regulate the hormones of obesity by using food and exercise.

You know you have to exercise, but you have no energy. Low thyroid and exhausted adrenals are two reasons you may gain weight and have no desire to work out. Buying a gym membership or a set of weights to use at home won't motivate you if you can't get off the sofa.

Low Thyroid Function

Low thyroid function (called hypothyroidism) affects approximately 20 to 25 percent of the population. And thyroid researchers believe an additional 10 to 20 percent may have suboptimal thyroid function—they have normal thyroid hormone blood tests but have many of the symptoms of low thyroid. Standard blood tests used in North America to determine low thyroid define "normal" too broadly. More women than men have low thyroid hormone levels. Low levels can lead to depression, dry skin, weight gain, inability to lose weight, lethargy and fatigue, sensitivity to temperature changes, recurrent infections, hair loss, and headaches. Low thyroid function makes you feel too tired to move. As mentioned earlier, thyroid hormones affect your body's metabolic rate. Your thyroid interacts closely with your adrenal glands, which sit above your kidneys. If the level of thyroid hormone is inadequate, the adrenals will become exhausted, and if the adrenals are exhausted, the thyroid will not manufacture enough thyroid hormone. It is a vicious cycle.

Exhausted Adrenal Glands

Adrenal exhaustion is a condition rarely discussed by medical doctors unless patients have a serious form of adrenal dysfunction called Addison's disease. The adrenal glands release sex hormones and stress-response hormones (cortisol), which help your body respond to stressors. Long-term elevations of cortisol can exhaust or wear out your adrenal glands. Women are especially prone to adrenal exhaustion now that they work full time while raising children and juggling many other demands. When your adrenal glands become impaired, your cortisol levels rise and stay elevated into the evening, preventing sleep or causing interrupted, very light sleep. High cortisol causes a drop in the hormones that regulate appetite and metabolism. By now you can probably see the connection between all the glands and hormones and how they can contribute to weight gain or weight loss. Chapter 4 will provide simple solutions to correct low thyroid function and weak adrenals, and includes self-tests for low thyroid function and weak adrenals.

Insulin: The Fat-Storage Hormone

Insulin, a hormone secreted by the pancreas, may be the main culprit contributing to your weight gain. Understanding how insulin functions can help you achieve your ideal weight and reduce the risk of developing heart disease, diabetes, or Syndrome X—a disorder marked by insulin resistance, glucose intolerance, weight gain, and abnormal blood fats. (These are explained in detail in Chapter 4.)

The standard North American diet is excessively high in bad carbohydrates and low in protein. Many of us combine this poor diet with a lack of exercise. The combination can disrupt the body's ability to regulate blood sugar adequately. In an effort to reduce the abnormally high blood sugar, the pancreas produces too much insulin, and then we gain weight, which causes our cells to become resistant to insulin and fat loss. Studies are proving that everyone who is overweight has some degree of insulin resistance, and insulin resistance puts us at higher risk of heart disease, cancers, and diabetes. Those with upper body fat (people who are shaped like apples) or who have excess weight around the middle are at serious risk of disease.

The Body Sense program takes this into account and provides solutions that will normalize blood sugar, insulin, and hormones. Thankfully, we can quickly improve our glucose/insulin actions and insulin resistance with just a few dietary modifications and the simple fitness techniques discussed in the following chapters.

3. Stress: The Cortisol Connection

Unrelenting chronic stress is another factor that promotes weight gain. New research shows that chronic stress causes your fat cells, especially those around the abdomen, to become resistant to fat loss. Cortisol, the stress hormone secreted by the adrenal glands, activates all fat cells to store fat! But central fat cells, found mainly in the abdominal wall, have four times the cortisol receptors on their cell membranes. Each time you are stressed, the cortisol fat mechanism turns on, and your body stores more fat to handle all the stress you are experiencing. Cortisol also increases in response to high insulin levels. Most of us contend with stress daily due to our fast-paced lifestyles. Stress is the single most costly claim in the workers' compensation system. Doctors Thomas Holmes and Richard Rahe, pioneering researchers in the field of stress, found the greater the number of life-changing events people experienced in a two-year period, the more frequently they became ill. Stress has surpassed the common cold as the most prevalent health problem in North America. Stress can be caused by constant noise, crowded cities with crime and pollution, negative emotions, depression, loneliness, unrealistic expectations, fear, and so much more. If you want to lose weight and keep it off, you must manage your cortisol levels effectively.

Serotonin: The Feel-Good Hormone

Serotonin, a neurotransmitter in the brain made from the amino acids found in proteins, tells your brain that your stomach is satisfied and that you can put down your fork. Neurotransmitters are messengers that communicate between cells. Low serotonin causes depression, lethargy, a preference for sugary foods, and ultimately obesity, because the brain senses it is starving. People who secrete too much cortisol have low serotonin levels, and these low levels may lead to problems in managing weight. Weight gain is a problem for most depressed people. When you diet and restrict protein-rich calories, your serotonin levels plummet.

17

Research on the connection between serotonin, cortisol, and weight gain has shown that lowering cortisol levels by managing stress and taking specific serotonin-enhancing nutritional supplements like 5-hydroxytryptophan (5-HTP) can help fight fat. (See Chapter 6 for more information on 5-HTP). This book provides solutions to normalize cortisol and other hormones, reduce stress, and get you on the road to an active lifestyle.

4. Food Choices

Most of the emphasis in weight loss is on the *quantity* of food, but the *quality* of the food you eat plays the most important role. Saturated fats, trans-fats, fake fats, artificial sweeteners, refined carbohydrates, processed meats and cheese, diet foods, and sodas conspire to make you fat and disrupt your hormones while increasing your risk of heart disease, diabetes, cancer, and other degenerative diseases. You may be eating chemically altered, toxic foods that clog your liver, disrupt your hormones, pollute your digestive tract, and starve you of healing nutrients. In Chapter 2, I discuss all the foods that make you slim and in Chapter 5 I give tips for treating food allergies and sensitivities. *The Body Sense Natural Diet* recommends only foods that are natural, rich in fiber and nutrients, free of pesticides and hormones, easy-to-prepare, and delicious.

Allergies and sensitivities to food also contribute to increased bloating, poor digestion, a disruption of the hormones in the digestive tract, weight gain, water retention, and an overall puffy appearance. Leaky gut syndrome is caused by years of food allergies, bacterial overgrowth in the digestive tract, candida yeast, and chronic stress (high cortisol). The term "leaky gut" refers to the waste, bacteria, and partially digested foods that are allowed to pass into the bloodstream from a damaged or leaky gut. The foreign substances that should stay in the digestive system float in the bloodstream, causing fluid retention and additional stress on the liver; some individuals gain about 10–15 lbs (4.5–7 kg) of extra fluids. Your body is approximately two-thirds water; this water is in all your cells and tissues where it is essential for all bodily functions. But when water becomes trapped in tissues and around cells, it can inhibit detoxification and proper cell function, including the movement of fat into and out of cells. Cellulite forms when your lymphatic system is overwhelmed by excess fluid retention and fat cell dysfunction. Chapter 8 includes cellulite busting solutions that work to eliminate existing cellulite and prevent further deposits.

5. Lack of Exercise

Exercise is essential, and a lack of it makes you fat, but first it is necessary to fix insulin, cortisol, serotonin, thyroid, and estrogen hormone imbalances; food allergies and sensitivities; and tired liver, thyroid, and adrenals, so when you start the exercise portion of the Body Sense program, you will get fast results, which will provide the incentive to stay committed to the program for life. See Chapter 7 for my fun, fast, and effective exercise program.

6. Liver Dysfunction

Perhaps you have been dieting for years and were never told that a healthy liver is essential for fat loss. The liver processes and packages your hormones, safely eliminates toxins, cleanses the blood of toxins, metabolizes proteins and carbohydrates into energy, manufactures cholesterol, breaks down fats, and performs many other vital functions.

You are bombarded with hundreds of toxins daily from the food you eat and drink, the air you breathe, and the internal chemicals that result from daily cellular processes. Therefore your liver must work nonstop to detoxify your body.

Estrogen Belly

The liver processes and packages your hormones and ensures healthy hormone balance. It also detoxifies excess estrogens or xenoestrogens (estrogens from the environment, found in plastics, pesticides, cosmetics, and hundreds of other common items, discussed in Chapter 8) that build up in the body and contribute to estrogen overload and increased fat storage.

Any disruption of the liver detoxification pathway contributes to excesses or imbalances in hormones. In particular, too much estrogen, also called "estrogen dominance," is one reason women have a difficult time losing fat around the abdominal area. It is also the reason men tend to develop a beer belly and breasts in their forties and beyond. A decreased rate of estrogen excretion contributes to what we commonly call "estrogen belly," too much fat around the middle. This is common in menopausal women.

Making Cholesterol

The liver also manufactures half of your body's cholesterol; the other half comes from the food you eat. Eighty percent of the cholesterol made by your liver is used to make bile. Every day the liver manufactures and secretes more than one quart (1L) of bile, which is stored in the gall-bladder for later use. Bile helps the digestion and assimilation of fats and fat-soluble vitamins and helps eliminate toxins from the body. Bile salts stimulate the secretion of water into the large intestine to help move waste products along, promoting healthy bowel movements.

Fatty Liver

Excess weight around the middle, fatty yellow bumps in the whites of the eyes, fatty cysts, and skin mottled with age spots are all signs of an overwhelmed or congested liver, commonly called a fatty liver. It is a result of clogged bile ducts, inadequate secretion of bile, or a liver overwhelmed or congested by too many toxins. Substances such as prescription drugs or alcohol can contribute to a fatty liver. Toxins, drugs, and alcohol cause our liver to inadequately break down or emulsify fats and our cells to store fat. The result is weight gain or resistance to fat loss.

Liver Stress Quiz

For each of the following, write the number 1 for mild symptoms, 2 for moderate, and 5 for severe:

___ You have chronic indigestion (heartburn, gas)

___ You have a distended abdomen (your abdomen sticks out either above or below your belly button)

___ You are constipated (you are not having one 12-inch (170mm) bowel movement or three 4-inch (55mm) bowel movements per day)

___ You have cellulite on your hips, thighs, buttocks, stomach, or arms

___ You have itchy skin, but no sign of rashes or lesions

___ You have eye problems (red, itchy, watery, or dry eyes, or spots in vision)

_____ You are fatigued, especially in the morning
_____ You have hot feet at night
_____ You suffer headaches and migraines
_____ You have insomnia or restless sleep
_____ You have menopausal symptoms or PMS
_____ You have muscle and/or joint pain
_____ You always feel tense in the neck and back
_____ You are angry or irritable
_____ You have depression or feel low
_____ You are stubborn
_____ You are negative
_____ You feel resentful
_____ **Total**

A score of more than 25 suggests a congested, stressed liver.

Because the liver is such a remarkable organ, involved in every function from metabolism to blood filtering, immunity, digestion, nutrient absorption, and hormone balance, a variety of symptoms can occur when it is not functioning at peak performance. In Chinese medicine, body organs are viewed as focal points for particular types of energy. The liver energy system governs the nervous system, the eyes, tendons, muscle tone, sexual energy, and motor activity in the body. The Chinese consider the liver to be the organ most strongly affected by emotions. When the liver is stressed by poor food, environmental toxins, or lack of sleep, anger, depression and irritability are more prevalent. You will learn in Chapter 3 that your emotions play havoc with your hormones, causing food cravings, binge eating, lack of control, and the secretion of too much cortisol, which all create liver stress. The liver is one organ in the body that heals rapidly when provided with the right food and nutrients. In Chapter 5 _The Body Sense Natural Diet_ provides the keys to rapid weight loss by quickly correcting liver imbalances.

7. Genetics

Genetics has been used as an excuse for weight problems. Yes, some of us have fat cells that respond differently and, yes, your mother and her mother may have been overweight, but these are not reasons for you to be overweight. Almost a decade ago, I read a book called *Your Family Tree Connection* by Chris Reading and Ross Meillon. This book left a lasting impression on me at a time when I was diligently studying genetics. The book undermined much of what I had learned. It gave clear evidence that nutritional deficiencies, allergies, and food sensitivities brought on by the way a family eats from generation to generation were a contributing factor to many genetically related conditions. Think about who taught you how to cook and the recipes you still use today. Were they passed down from generation to generation? And were the people in these generations overweight? This is especially important for women because our moms teach us how to cook and we often continue these cooking and eating patterns. Males move into another family with its own unique set of foods and recipes, which could be good or bad for the waistline. A genetic predisposition to obesity does not mean you have to become obese. It just means you have to eat differently than the previous generations of your family. Once you alter the types of food you eat and correct your metabolism and hormonal imbalance, weight management will be effortless, not the constant struggle you are used too.

LOOKING FORWARD

You may have endured the no-fat, low-fat, high-protein, low-carbohydrate, grapefruit, blood type, or other diet of the month with very good intentions but without success. The restriction and deprivation recommended in most diets ultimately cause dieters to fear food. This, combined with the aggressive marketing and advertising by manufacturers of low-fat, no-fat, and reduced-fat food, leave people unsure of what to eat. I trust that when you finish reading this book, you will realize you can eat the foods suggested and adopt the strategies because they fit into your new lifestyle, which will be one of energy and vitality. The book will open the door to a new you. You will no longer have a fear of food; instead, you will discover the missing key in your personal weight loss battle. It may be low thyroid, too much estrogen, not enough happy hormones, adrenal exhaustion, liver congestion, or some of the other factors I discuss. Food will become your friend because you will know which foods turn on certain hormones and which ones turn them off, making weight loss effortless.

Exercise will no longer be a chore as you learn that it can enhance the action of the foods you eat and flip the switch on your metabolism, sending it into fat-burning mode. *The Body Sense Natural Diet* program will put you in charge of your health and help you discover that beautiful body you have always wanted. Those men and women who have been following this program for the last two years have told me they have never looked back. They now eat for success and have gained new health and a vibrancy that was missing before they changed their lives. This book is packed with health-improvement tips, not just fat-loss suggestions.

chapter two

Tell Me How Right Now

I know you want to get started on your new eating plan today. This chapter will launch into the program, providing shopping lists, meal plans, and everything else you need to get going right away. The rest of the chapters will explain all the supporting evidence for long-term weight management and the prevention and treatment of the diseases associated with being overweight. Today you are one day closer to your ideal body.

The Body Sense Natural Diet is designed to achieve a new you in six weeks—forty-two days. You are not going to count fat grams or calories, but you will keep track of the number of servings of good healthy foods you eat every day—and you must eat. Starving and binge dieting make us fat by lowering our metabolic rate. You are also not going to weigh yourself during the entire six weeks. You can weigh yourself at the start and again at the end, but you are going to rely more on your body measurements as an indicator of success. Take a photo of yourself before starting the program and another in six weeks. If you are really brave, wear a bathing suit or shorts and a T-shirt for the photo. Your goal is to transform your body. I'll be asking you to take some measurements—key indicators of the shape you're in right now. You'll come back to this section in six weeks to chart your progress and to see how you've changed.

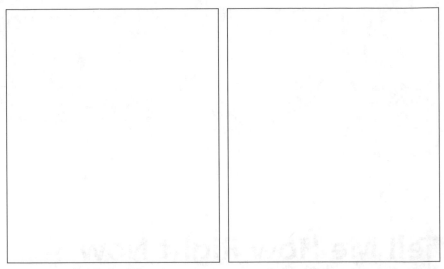

Tape your before photo here   Tape your after photo here

Body measurements	before	after
Arm midway between elbow and armpit:		
Bust/chest:		
Waist:		
Hips:		
Thigh midway between knee and crotch:		

The thousands of people who have followed the Body Sense Natural Diet program rave about its benefits. The thing participants like best about this plan is that they don't feel hungry and started to lose inches in the first few weeks. The program is so effective you will want to exercise to speed up the process of uncovering the new you under that layer of extra padding. You don't count calories, fat grams, or anything else, so you are not constantly thinking about food. After six weeks, your metabolic rate and appetite will be reset and you will start to metabolize foods properly. You will have boundless energy and vitality. Finally, your blood sugar and cholesterol levels will normalize.

BUILDING YOUR SHOPPING LIST

Before you visit the grocery and health food stores, clear your cupboards and refrigerator of unhealthy foods. If you have cookies, crackers, and sweets in your pantry, you will be tempted, but if they are not in the house, you can't eat them. Get rid of that freezer full of white bread and ice cream. Bad carbohydrates cause cravings that provoke hunger by stimulating the secretion of insulin. Protein and good fats make you feel satisfied, and you will no longer constantly reach for something to eat. When you are hungry, you want to have the proper foods at your fingertips, so make a shopping list that includes the foods suggested below. Visit the grocery and health food stores before you embark on this new eating plan. If you have never been into a health food store, you are in for a treat. Some stores sell organic food along with food supplements and beauty products. Also look in the phone book for a company that delivers organic foods. If you don't find one, ask at the health food store if they know of one in your area. It is not imperative that you eat organic, but now that you are going to be eating in the healthiest way possible, why not eat organically grown foods as well? Make sure you purchase an abundance of the right foods.

SLIMMING FOODS AND SUPPLEMENTS

The following are recommendations. As there are thousands of foods, it is impossible to list them all here. You can also use the glycemic index food list as a source of food choices. Remember to choose foods low on the glycemic index. The lower the foods are on the chart, the faster you will lose weight. For the first few weeks, the Body Sense Diet program focuses on foods below 20 on the chart. Choosing foods below 20 will ensure a jump start in your weight loss goals. You want to see results quickly, and if you choose foods below 20, you will. After the first two weeks, foods below 60 on the chart can be added to provide variety. Remember the goal is to learn how to eat to maintain optimal health for life, not just for 42 days. Choose foods that are in their natural state, and eat organic foods whenever possible. Avoid all foods containing sugar, artificial sweeteners, trans-fatty acids (you will see them listed on the label as hydrogenated and partially hydrogenated), and processed foods.

Protein
❑ bison
❑ canned water-packed wild salmon
❑ dairy products
❑ free-range chicken and turkey (breasts, ground lean breast)
❑ free-range eggs and/or omega-3-enriched eggs
❑ grassland-fed beef
❑ kefir (kefir contains friendly bacteria yogurt doesn't have, and it recolonizes the intestinal tract with good bacteria)
❑ lamb
❑ lobster or crab (canned water-packed)
❑ organic fermented soy protein powder
❑ organic tofu (soft or firm)
❑ ostrich
❑ protein powder (whey, fermented soy, pea, or rice)
❑ sardines
❑ scallops
❑ shrimp
❑ organic sour cream
❑ tuna (fresh, or canned water-packed)
❑ venison
❑ wild fish (cod, bass, haddock, halibut, mackerel, perch, pollack, snapper, sole, trout, whitefish)

Nuts and Seeds
❑ almonds
❑ Brazil nuts
❑ filberts
❑ flaxseeds
❑ pecans
❑ sesame seeds
❑ sunflower seeds
❑ walnuts

Good Carbohydrates
Fruits
❑ blackberries
❑ blueberries (fresh, frozen unsweetened)
❑ cherries (fresh, canned unsweetened)
❑ cranberries (fresh, frozen unsweetened)
❑ dried apricots
❑ kiwi
❑ lemons and limes (or their pure juice only, no concentrates)
❑ peaches and pears (fresh or packed in their own juice)
❑ plums
❑ raspberries (fresh, frozen unsweetened)
❑ unsweetened cranberry juice (no concentrates)
❑ unsweetened grapefruit juice (no concentrates)
❑ watermelon

Choose other fruits from the glycemic index list.

Vegetables

❑ arugula
❑ avocado
❑ Brussels sprouts
❑ broccoli
❑ cauliflower
❑ celery
❑ chard
❑ cucumber
❑ eggplant
❑ kale
❑ lettuces
❑ mushrooms
❑ purple cabbage
❑ rhubarb
❑ scallions
❑ seed sprouts of all kinds
❑ zucchini

Any vegetable is acceptable except white potatoes, corn (canned baby corn in moderation is allowed as their starches are reduced), parsnips, pumpkin, beets, and carrots. Even lactic acid–fermented sauerkraut is excellent for digestion. Olives packed in their own oil or water are especially important for those with adrenal fatigue.

Starches, Breads, Crackers, and Chips
The following are allowed only after the first two weeks of the program.
❏ unsweetened, protein-enriched, whole-grain rye and pumpernickel breads
❏ tortillas

See other acceptable foods on the glycemic index chart.

Beans and Legumes
❏ black beans
❏ chickpeas
❏ lentils
❏ pinto beans
❏ split peas
❏ white navy beans

Breakfast Cereal
❏ steel-cut, large rolled oats (not quick cooking or instant)
❏ ground flaxseeds
❏ 7-grain cereal
❏ unsweetened all bran cereal

Pasta
❏ cheese tortellini or ravioli (meat filled)
❏ real egg fettuccini
❏ whole-grain pastas

Good Dairy Products
❏ organic cheese
❏ organic milk
❏ organic yogurt, unsweetened and unflavored

Soups (canned)
❏ black bean
❏ lentil
❏ tomato

Sweeteners
❏ stevia
❏ xylitol

Avoid all synthetic sweeteners and glucose or any sugar ending in -ose, such as dextrose, lactose, and fructose.

Fats and Oils

☐ cold-pressed organic flaxseed, sunflower, pistachio, or pumpkin seed oil for dressings

☐ extra virgin olive oil or sesame oil for cooking

☐ organic coconut butter (excellent for cooking; provides medium-chain triglycerides, which improve thyroid function and aid fat loss by maintaining blood sugar)

Condiments and Spices

☐ balsamic vinegar

☐ capers

☐ cardamom

☐ carob or cocoa powder

☐ cayenne

☐ chives

☐ cilantro

☐ cinnamon

☐ coriander

☐ garlic

☐ mayonnaise

☐ organic apple cider vinegar

☐ peppercorns

☐ real flavor extracts, no sugar added (vanilla, anise, almond, lemon, etc.)

☐ rosemary

☐ sage

☐ sea salt

☐ thyme

☐ turmeric

☐ unsweetened Dijon mustard

☐ unsweetened salsa

Tea and Coffee

❑ herbal teas (unsweetened) throughout the day
❑ organic coffee 1 cup (250 mL per day)

NUTRITIONAL SUPPLEMENTS

Multivitamins with minerals are the foundation of your weight-loss program. Purchase a good-quality multivitamin with mineral supplement. It is impossible to get all your nutrient requirements from the foods you eat. Your food is grown on soils depleted of nutrients, picked before it is ripe and shipped hundreds of miles before you purchase it. Most people do not eat 7 to 10 half-cup servings of fruits and vegetables—the basic amount needed to get the minimum requirement of nutrients. A one-a-day vitamin pill will not have enough of the nutrients you need for proper nutrient support and optimal health. Ensure the supplement you buy contains at least 30 mg of each B vitamin, 1000 mg of vitamin C, 200 mg of vitamin E, and all these minerals: zinc, magnesium, chromium, selenium, potassium, manganese, and calcium. See the resource section for vitamin and mineral recommendations.

Throughout this book I may recommend other nutritional supplements for a certain disease or condition, such as diabetes, or health concern, such as constipation, adrenal stress, estrogen overload, or cellulite. The shopping list will get you started on the program. As you proceed you may need to support your weight loss program with other supplements

Aids for Digestion

To ensure that your body is breaking down and absorbing the foods you eat, you need digestive aids. After decades of eating processed foods, and due to aging your digestion becomes impaired. To support proper breakdown of the foods you eat, purchase a good-quality, plant-based digestive enzyme. You'll find this at your local health food store or in the nutrient section of a pharmacy or grocery store. Follow the directions on the label, which will generally tell you to take 2 capsules 15 minutes before each meal. Immediately you will notice that you do not have gas, bloating, and burping after a meal, and within days your bowel movements will improve. See Chapter 5 for more information on digestive aids.

- plant-based digestive enzymes
- Swedish bitters digestive aid

Protein Powders

Protein powder is an essential part of your weight-loss program. Find a brand that tastes delicious, as you will be using the powder as a snack or meal supplement often throughout the day. Protein powders come from many sources, including whey, fermented soy, peas, and rice. If you are not allergic to dairy products, whey protein provides the highest biological value of protein. Many whey protein powders are lactose reduced, and some lactose-intolerant individuals can eat them without symptoms. If you choose soy protein make sure it is not genetically modified and is organic. I prefer fermented soy protein, which is much easier to digest, as the protein is predigested and offers many health benefits (see Chapter 6 for more information on protein powders). Whatever type of protein you choose, make sure it tastes great, or you won't want to use it. Pick a plain flavor to add to cooked foods and flavored varieties to enhance yogurt and other bland-tasting foods.

Metabolism Boosts/Fat, Carb and Sugar Blockers

You may not need fat-burning supplements, but people who have been dieting for years often need some help in boosting their metabolism or blocking the absorption of the occasional fattening food. Green tea extract, cayenne, bitter orange, yerba maté, and ginger root are powerful thermogenics, which can help burn fat faster by enhancing your metabolism. Look for metabolism boosters containing these ingredients at the health food store.

Purchase Cassia nomame, a herb that inhibits the absorption of saturated fats by about 30 percent. Also buy Phase II, an extract from the white kidney bean (extensive studies show that it blocks starch absorption) and gymnema extract, a herb that helps your body metabolize sugar. See Chapter 6 for details about the research into these herbs and supplements and how they work to help burn fat.

Low Thyroid Function

You learned in Chapter 1 that it's hard to lose weight if you have low thyroid function. I recommend the following herbs and nutrients to support healthy thyroid function:

- L-tyrosine (an amino acid)
- Ashwagandha (*Withania somnifera*)
- *Commiphora mukul* (Guggal)
- Potassium iodide

You also need the supporting nutrients found in your multivitamin, and minerals copper and manganese, plus pantothenic acid. If you are on thyroid medication but continue to have low thyroid symptoms these nutrients can be taken safely along with your thyroid medication. Do not stop your medication. The nutrients are to be used in conjunction with your thyroid medication. Have a thyroid hormone test (TSH, T4, T3, and thyroid antibodies) about 6 weeks after you start taking the nutrients; some individuals do not require as much thyroid medicine when they are taking the nutrients.

If you have suboptimal thyroid function, take the nutrients to support thyroid health. See Chapter 4 for a detailed explanation of low thyroid and the actions of the nutrients. Do not use these nutrients if you have hyperthyroid (overactive thyroid). Overactive thyroid, a serious condition, affects a small percentage of the population.

Diabetes

Go to Chapter 9 and read all about this condition before visiting the supermarket and health food store.

FOOD, GLORIOUS FOOD

Food is the cornerstone of the Body Sense Natural Diet. When you shop, look for foods that are organic, fresh, unsweetened, not genetically modified, free of hydrogenated or partially hydrogenated fats, and without aspartame or sucralose. Beware of the inner aisles of the grocery store, where the processed, packaged, and fattening foods are. The outer aisles usually store the fresh fruits and vegetables, the meat and dairy products, bulk foods, frozen foods, and the baked goods. Become a label reader. Don't buy items if you can't understand the labels or if you don't know what the ingredients are.

LOW GLYCEMIC INDEX FOODS

It is so simple to be healthier, thinner, and more energetic once you learn which foods to avoid and which to choose. People with diabetes, obesity, cancer, and heart disease who choose low glycemic index foods (below 60) will find that many of their symptoms quickly heal. Low glycemic foods balance blood sugar, lower insulin requirements, reduce body fat, reduce blood pressure, improve the immune system, promote longevity, and provide overall enhanced well-being. The Body Sense program does not eliminate or drastically reduce carbohydrates. This diet focuses on good, healthy carbohydrates that have a low glycemic index rating.

For the most complete listing of foods, see www.mendosa.com and view the extensive glycemic index chart. David Mendosa is a medical journalist, and he has an extremely interesting Web site, especially for those who are overweight or have diabetes. The foods I have chosen for the program are low glycemic index foods. Just think natural, as Mother Nature intended. Choose foods that are whole foods, not processed, that are protein-enriched, and that are without sugar or fake fats.

GLYCEMIC INDEX

Avoid foods between 100 and 60

Food	Glycemic Index
Glucose	100
Potato, baked	98
Carrots, cooked	92
White rice, instant	91
Cornflakes	92
Honey	74
Bread, white	72
Bagels	72
Melba toast	70
Potato, mashed	70

Bread, wheat	69
Table sugar	65
Beets	64
Raisins	61
Bran muffin	60

Eat foods rated 60 or less in moderation.

Pita	57
Oatmeal, large cut (not instant)	55
Popcorn (air popped)	55
Buckwheat	54
Banana	53
Brown rice	50
Grapefruit juice, unsweetened	48
Bread, whole-grain pumpernickel	46
Soy milk	44
Bread, dark whole-grain rye	42
Pinto beans	42
Whole-grain pasta	41
Apples	39
Tomato juice, canned unsweetened	38
All-bran cereal ™	38
Tomatoes	38
Yogurt, plain	38
Yams	37
Chickpeas	36
Skim milk	32
Strawberries*	32
Real egg fettuccine	32
Kidney beans	29
Whole-grain spaghetti, protein enriched	27
Peaches	26
Cherries	24
Fructose (Limit consumption; although fructose is a low GI food, it has problems.)	20

*Strawberries are very heavily sprayed with pesticides. Buy only organic.

Foods below 20 can be eaten freely

Non-starchy vegetables are below 20 on the glycemic index:

Arugula

Asparagus

Avocado

Broccoli

Brussels sprouts

Cauliflower

Celery

Chard

Cucumber

Eggplant

Kale

Lettuces

Mushrooms

Purple cabbage

Rhubarb

Scallions

Seed sprouts

Zucchini

Meat, poultry, fish, eggs, fats, and oils are not rated because they have almost no carbohydrates.

CARBOHYDRATES, FATS, AND PROTEINS

The three main nutrients of food are protein, carbohydrates, and fats, and all are used as fuel for the body. But protein and fats are the main sources of fuel used for repair, maintenance, and growth of all cells in the body. Carbohydrates provide us with quick energy but are not necessary for survival; protein and fats can be used as a substitute for carbohydrates. For example, the Inuit traditional diet lived on fat and protein, but no carbohydrates. When people go on carbohydrate-free diets but do not get adequate good fats they end up feeling depressed, they have no energy, and they get the shakes because they are not getting the fats they need for adequate brain and nervous system function. If there are lots of carbohydrates in your diet, your body will burn these first and stop burning fats.

When carbohydrates are present in abundance, your body also converts them to fat, especially if you are not doing enough exercise to burn off the carbohydrates you are eating. To burn fat, choose the low glycemic carbohydrates in small quantities and eat more protein and good fat. Then your body will burn fat faster.

What Is a Carbohydrate?

Carbohydrates supply your body with energy. Your body converts all carbohydrates, with the exception of fiber, into glucose, a major source of fuel. Found predominantly in plant foods and, to a lesser extent, in milk and milk products, carbohydrates are divided into two groups: complex carbohydrates, which are made up of hundreds of sugar molecules linked together, and simple carbohydrates, which usually contain up to three sugar molecules. Simple carbohydrates are most often identified by their sweet taste and are found in refined and processed foods.

Simple carbohydrates include fructose (fruit sugar), sucrose (table sugar), and lactose (milk sugar). Fruit, although a simple carbohydrate, is allowed in the diet in its whole, natural state. Avoid fruit juices that no longer contain the fiber are to be avoided (except for lemon and lime juice, which help slow the digestion of starches, thus lowering the glycemic index of foods).

Complex carbohydrates include fiber and starches, which are found in vegetables, legumes, beans, nuts, seeds, and whole, unrefined grains. Fiber, found in plants, is another source of carbohydrates. Although you don't digest it, fiber is an important carbohydrate for sweeping the colon, thus preventing constipation; it also lowers blood sugar, cholesterol, and triglycerides.

The worst form of carbohydrate is the refined type found in cookies, cakes, crackers, and desserts. Refined carbohydrates offer empty calories and give you no vitamins and minerals. Increase the number of complex carbohydrates you eat, and reduce the refined carbohydrates. If everyone stopped eating all white pasta, white rice, white flour, and white sugar, diabetes, high blood pressure, high cholesterol, and cancer rates would drop dramatically.

Within the complex carbohydrate category, there are foods that affect the rate of insulin release into the bloodstream. Too much insulin or too fast a release of insulin has health consequences and is linked to the development of diabetes, obesity, and increased aging, so choose foods below 60 on the glycemic index.

Lots of vegetables (good carbohydrates) form the basis of the Body Sense eating plan, especially the cruciferous vegetables: broccoli, Brussels sprouts, cauliflower, kale, and cabbage. The nutrients in these vegetables help keep your liver healthy; they aid fat loss by detoxifying excess estrogens; and they provide bulk to eliminate constipation. This program is not devoid of all carbohydrates, but is based on good carbohydrates that do not cause a rapid rise in blood sugar and have a glycemic index of 60 or lower. Vegetables, most of which have a GI below 20 include non-starchy vegetables such as leafy greens, celery, broccoli, asparagus, avocado, tomatoes, and sprouts.

Fat Phobia

Every dieter I have counseled is terrified of eating fat. We have been trained by dieticians and diet support groups to use cooking sprays on the frying pan and search labels for the words "no fat." When food companies remove fats from foods, they often replace the fats with sugar. So although the food may be non-fat, it has hundreds of calories of sugars or contain fake sugars that disrupt the body's chemistry. Fat makes your body feel satisfied and is essential to healthy brain function. Fat is the most concentrated source of energy for your body. Without the right kinds of fat in your diet, your hair will fall out, your thyroid gland will not function well, you will become depressed, and you will eat more and get fatter. So repeat after me: "The right fats can make me slim. The right fats unlock fat stored in my fat cells. The right fats will increase my rate of metabolism." Repeat this until you believe it. Think about giving your body good, clean sources of fat from foods like nuts and seeds and their oils. You would not fuel your car with dirty gasoline, yet every day you pollute your body with toxic fats in the form of margarines, processed oils, trans fats (see below for information on trans fats), shortenings, and lards, all of which contribute to your health problems.

Understanding Fat

When you consume fat the gastrointestinal tract breaks it down into the triglyceride form, into free fatty acids. The fatty acids, derived from saturated fats found in red meat and dairy products, are the main source of energy production and fat storage in the body. When you eat too much saturated fat, then couple it with an inactive lifestyle, you gain weight. A diet that contains higher amounts of the good fats found in healthy, cold-pressed, organic oils such as flaxseed, hemp, sunflower, safflower, evening primrose, and borage, discourages fat storage and encourages fat burning.

Saturated Fats—the Good, the Bad and the Not-So-Bad

Saturated fats are semisolid at room temperature and are found in animal products (such as red meat, pork, lamb, and lard) and dairy products (milk, cheese, and butter), as well as in processed foods. They are generally considered "bad" fats as they can contribute to heart disease; therefore, most health authorities recommend a reduction of saturated fats in the diet.

However, not all saturated fats are created equal. There are three subgroups of saturated fats that are characterized by the length of their fat chain: short-chain, medium-chain, and long-chain fats.

The Good Saturates

Short-chain saturates—found in butter, coconut oil, and palm kernel oil—do not clog arteries, nor do they cause heart disease. Rather, they are easily digested and a source of fuel for energy. As well, short-chain saturates do not contain as many calories as the longer-chain fatty acids. Butter is only 80 percent fat, and margarine is 100 percent fat, so 1 lb (.5 kg) of butter has 8 fewer calories than the same amount of margarine made with seed oils.

The Not-So-Bad Saturates

Medium-chain saturates are found in several different foods, but the highest content (just as in short-chain saturates) is also found in palm kernel and coconut oils, and they are not associated with increasing cholesterol levels or the occurrence of heart disease. Medium-chain triglyceride oils (MCT oils) are used in special medical formulas for people who need energy from fat but have trouble digesting it from regular dietary sources, and for athletes and dieters who want to convert fat into energy rather than store it as fat.

The Bad Saturates

Long-chain saturates are the "bad" fats associated with raising LDL (the bad cholesterol), lowering HDL (the good cholesterol), and increasing the risk of heart disease. The bad saturated fats are those found in red meat, including beef, veal, lamb, ham, and pork. So you want to eat these foods in moderation. Long-chain saturates are also a by-product of hydrogenation, a process that turns a liquid fat (at room temperature) into a solid and is employed in the manufacture of most margarines and shortening. Long-chain saturates are also abundantly present in restaurant fried foods, junk food, packaged baked goods, and processed foods. Hydrogenation or partial hydrogenation also distorts the fatty acids into a more poisonous form.

The Deadly Fats

The deadliest fats are trans-fatty acids. These fats are formed when high temperatures and hydrogenation turn refined oils into margarines, shortenings, and partially hydrogenated vegetable oils to make them solid or semisolid, thus giving them a longer shelf life. Trans-fatty acids damage your cardiovascular system, promote cancer, impair immune function, and more. Trans fats are found in all fast foods, potato chips, french fries, baby biscuits, breakfast cereals, cookies, microwave popcorn, and some margarines, to name just a few. All the oils used in commercially produced salad dressings also contain trans fats as a result of the high heat process used to make these oils shelf stable. Barbecuing, blackening, or high-heat frying foods creates trans fats, as well. Eliminate trans fats. Not only do they contribute to obesity and weight gain, they also destroy your health. Use coconut butter instead of lard and shortening. Don't eat margarine. Choose healthy oils that are cold-pressed and organic (found in the whole foods section of your grocery store or in a health food store). Use olive oil, sesame oil, or coconut butter for low-heat sautéing; for salad dressings use flaxseed oil, hempseed oil, walnut oil, olive oil, sunflower oil, pumpkin seed oil, or macadamia nut oil; for baking use sunflower oil, butter, or coconut butter. Do not fry foods: frying promotes free radicals, which promote cancer and heart disease.

Scientists have stated that trans-fatty acids are almost twice as bad as saturated fats in terms of the damage they cause to your cardiovascular system. Health Canada and the U.S. Food and Drug Administration have implemented new regulations requiring all pre-packaged foods to list the trans fat content by 2006, and eventually these regulations will be applicable to the fast-food industry so that you will know the trans fat content of your fries and doughnut.

Numerous research studies have shown that trans fats are more damaging to the heart than saturated fats. And the Institute of Medicine, a division of the U.S. National Academy of Science, released a report in July 2002 on trans fats. It is a strongly worded report declaring that there are no safe levels of trans fats and that consumption should be reduced as much as possible. The institute declined to declare any upper limits on trans fats.

Trans-fatty acids are man-made—that is, artificial. Your body cannot recognize them as nutrients and therefore cannot process them. There has been much debate over whether saturated or trans fats are worse. But remember: harmful trans fats do not occur naturally. Saturated fats do. The Harvard School of Public Health has declared trans fats dangerous to health. While saturated fats in high levels are not healthy for the body either, they are still a source of energy that your body can use. Trans fats are truly junk food and should be avoided. Hydrogenated or partially hydrogenated oils in food-product ingredient lists means that the product contains trans fats.

Alberto Ascherio, the lead researcher on a team from the Harvard School of Public Health and the Wageningen Centre for Food Sciences in the Netherlands, published a review in the June 1999 issue of *New England Journal of Medicine*, stating that "Coronary heart disease (CHD) kills 500,000 Americans each year. According to our estimations, if trans fats were replaced by unsaturated vegetable oils, we would expect to see at least 30,000 fewer persons die prematurely from CHD each year."

University of Maryland researchers confirm earlier estimates that the average American consumes at least 12 g or approximately half an ounce per day of trans fats, which adds up to approximately 22 cups (5280 mL) of trans fats per year. Statistics Canada reports that Canadians are eating 24 lbs (10.75 kg) of trans fat–loaded shortening every year, up from 18 lbs (8.2 kg) in 1987. To put that into perspective, that is twenty-four 1-lb (.5 kg) blocks of shortening.

In 2003 McDonald's™ and Kraft Foods™ both vowed to make their products healthier. Why after all these years? McDonald's had reduced earnings for the first time in their fifty-year history, and when they researched why their revenue had dropped, they discovered that it was because people are eating healthier foods. Kraft reached similar conclusions and decided they should take some responsibility for helping North Americans lose a few pounds. They formed a panel of health and nutrition experts to review all their products and recommend solutions. The panel will look at total calories, fat, saturated fat, cholesterol, sugar, salt, and especially trans-fatty acids. Kraft wants to eliminate all trans fats or cut them to a half a gram per serving in their cookies and cakes. Although I applaud fast-food companies for recognizing the need to provide healthier foods, the timing seems a bit suspicious in the wake of the new labeling laws. The governments in both Canada and the United States have mandated labeling of foods containing trans fats. Large food manufacturers have to reduce or eliminate the trans fats because the numbers will be right there on the label for you to see. If you knew that the baby biscuits for your cherished infant were high in deadly trans fats, you would not purchase them. Food manufacturers know this. My concern is what they will use to replace the hydrogenated oils they are currently using. In the past, manufacturers of no-fat, low-fat foods replaced fat with sugars. We don't want to trade one evil for another.

Very Good Unsaturated Fats

Unsaturated fats are liquid at room temperature and are generally considered to be "good" fats. Typically, the more liquid a fat is, the healthier it is. Unsaturated fats can be further classified as either monounsaturated or polyunsaturated. Monounsaturated fats remain liquid at room temperature, but solidify in colder temperatures. Sources of these fatty acids are olive, canola, and peanut oils. These fatty acids are associated with the good cholesterol. I do not recommend canola, because it is genetically modified rapeseed. It is found abundantly in grocery store salad dressings and spreads. Peanut oil is also not recommended, as it is heavily refined. Extra-virgin olive oil is the recommended oil. Do not purchase light olive oil, as it has been processed to remove the good fats.

Polyunsaturated fats remain liquid at room temperature and remain liquid even in colder temperatures. Sources of polyunsaturated fats include black currant oil, borage oil, corn oil, flaxseed oil, safflower oil, sesame oil, soy oil, sunflower oil, evening primrose oil, and fatty fish. Black currant, borage, and evening primrose oils are sold in capsules, and the other oils are available as liquids.

Unsaturated fats can also be further classified as omega-3, omega-6, or omega-9. The omega-3s and omega-6s are polyunsaturated and are essential because your body cannot make them. The omega-9s are monounsaturated and non-essential because your body can make them from other fatty acids.

The Truth about Coconut Oil

Coconut oil has been wrongly branded as a nutritional evil since the 1960s, when data collected from research were misinterpreted, concluding that coconut oil raised blood cholesterol levels. In fact, it was the omission of essential fatty acids in the experimental diet that caused the observed health problems, not the inclusion of the coconut oil. Coconut oil is a short-chain fat that is easily digested and used by the body. More recent subject groups studied in the South Pacific for their regular use of coconut oil in the diet exhibited low incidences of coronary artery disease and low serum cholesterol levels. Little or no change is evident in serum cholesterol levels when an EFA-rich diet contains non-hydrogenated saturated fats. Coconut oil also supports healthy thyroid function. It is naturally saturated, so it does not need to go through hydrogenation (an unhealthy process that changes oils into a solid or semisolid state). It becomes harder as it is exposed to lower temperatures. Coconut oil has other benefits: it is slightly lower in calories than most other fats and oils, and you don't need to use as much coconut oil as you would other oils when cooking or baking.

Coconut-Flaxseed Spread Recipe

1/2 cup	flaxseed oil	125 mL
1 cup	coconut butter	250 mL

Place flaxseed oil in freezer for two hours or more. Melt coconut butter on low temperature. Remove from heat. Add frozen flaxseed oil. Blend and keep in the refrigerator for up to six weeks. Store in an opaque container to prolong life. Do not use for cooking or baking. It can be used as a spread in place of butter and margarine. Makes 1-1/2 cups (375 mL).

Butter Is Better

The great debate over whether butter is better than margarine still exists, and it is a travesty that butter has been unfairly demonized. Fats and oils experts, including Mary Enig, author of *Know Your Fats*, believe that butter is an important fat and one that should not be replaced by hydrogenated fats like margarine. Butter contains many healthful components, including lecithin, which helps your body break down cholesterol. It is also a rich source of vitamin A, which is necessary for the healthy functioning of the adrenal and thyroid glands. The vitamins A and E and the mineral selenium in butter also serve as important antioxidants in protecting against free radical damage that can destroy tissues and weaken artery walls.

Butter is made from cream and contains a wide range of short- and medium-chain fatty acids, as well as monounsaturated and some polyunsaturated fatty acids. The dangers of butter's saturated fat components have been blown out of proportion; remember, not all saturated fats are equal.

Natural saturated fatty acids like coconut oil and butter have vital and protective properties. While it is important to limit excess consumption of saturated fats, especially the long-chain ones found in red meat, a balanced diet should contain the beneficial saturated fats found in butter and coconut oil.

Butter is one of the few foods available in our supermarkets that still contains natural conjugated linoleic acid (an essential fatty acid with fat-burning and cancer-fighting properties. For more information see Chapter 6.)

Your Fat Furnace

I will talk about thermogenesis, white fat, and brown fat throughout the book, so an explanation of what they are is in order. Thermogenesis is the creation of heat in your body. The food you eat provides you with energy, which is measured in calories. When your body burns calories (regardless of whether it is from sleeping or running a marathon), heat is produced. White fat is the insulating layer of fat just beneath the skin that buffers you from the cold and stores calories. This is the fat you so desperately try to get rid of. Brown fat surrounds your organs, cushioning the blood vessels and spinal column. You can't see brown fat on you. This is the type of fat

	Better Butter Recipe	
1 lb	butter	0.5 kg
1 cup	high-quality essential fatty acid–rich oil	250 mL
	(such as flaxseed oil, or any other organic, cold-pressed oil)	

Cut butter into eight pieces. Put butter and oil into the food processor and blend until smooth. Spoon into covered container and refrigerate. Not only will you have better butter, but it will remain soft even though refrigerated. Makes 2 cups (500 mL).

that is burned in the body to create heat, not the kind that stores calories. In other words, thermogenesis describes the activity of brown fat.

Thermogenesis is important for two functions: to burn calories and to adapt to cold. The ability of some animals to hibernate during the winter is due to thermogenesis. Their bodies burn brown fat to create heat. The heat, in addition to keeping them warm, burns the white fat for energy (to nourish their bodies even though they haven't eaten). You may have noticed that after eating a large steak, you start to sweat. This is called diet-induced thermogenesis. A portion of the food you eat is converted into heat, and the rest is metabolized, absorbed, and stored. During the conversion of food into useful substances, calories are burned, stimulating an increase in heat production. Research has shown that if you eat a meal of mostly protein, you can raise your fat-burning rate by more than 25 percent, and the rate will stay that high for six to eight hours. Carbohydrates (especially high-glycemic index or highly processed bad carbohydrates) increase thermogenesis by less than 10 percent, and this increase lasts for less than an hour. Thermogenesis and brown fat activity explain why it appears as if one person can eat all day without gaining an ounce while another person can gain weight just thinking about food. Thin people have activated brown fat, while overweight individuals have dormant brown fat. Some research has suggested that essential fatty acids, such as borage oil or evening primrose oil (sold in capsules), can stimulate brown fat activity and help burn white fat.

Certain essential fatty acids help increase thermogenesis, increasing metabolism and decreasing fat storage, thus helping prevent weight gain. Fatty acids released into the blood from fat stores or from dietary fat sources are used by the body to break down fats to be used for energy to create heat. They also help burn fat rather than store fat. By adding essential fatty acids from the food supplements evening primrose oil and borage oil to the diet, you can prompt your cells to create heat and thereby burn fat.

Protein

Your body requires twenty essential amino acids to facilitate the production of protein for cellular repair, the manufacture of hormones, immune system factors, enzymes, and tissues. Of those twenty amino acids, twelve can be made within the body, and the remaining eight must be obtained from food.

Two groups of proteins are found in your diet. Complete proteins—including meat, fish, poultry, cheese, eggs, milk, tofu, fermented soy, and whey protein powder—contain all the essential amino acids. Incomplete proteins—including grains, legumes, and leafy green vegetables—do not contain all the essential amino acids.

Some people have greater protein requirements than others. If you are very active, exercise strenuously, or do heavy labor, or if you are pregnant, you will need more protein than a couch potato. When choosing your protein sources, opt for free-range poultry and eggs, and wild fish over farm-grown fish, to avoid contamination from antibiotics and growth hormones. Purchase nuts in the shell and buy organic whenever you can. Protein is a big part of the Body Sense Natural Diet program. It is important not to choose toxic foods like bologna and hot dogs as your protein sources.

Exercise Category	Recommended Daily Protein Intake
	(Gg/lb)
Sedentary	0.36
Moderate	0.36–0.5
Endurance	0.5–0.8
Strength	0.6–0.8
Teenage	0.6–0.9

(Source: Leslie Beck, *The Complete Idiot's Guide to Total Nutrition for Canadians*. Toronto: Prentice-Hall Canada, 2000.)

A protein-rich breakfast will jump-start your metabolism, revving up your fat-burning furnace by 25 percent and keeping it that way for up to eight hours. The classic cereal and skim milk breakfast does not accomplish this. Protein powders, free-range red meats, eggs, chicken, wild fish, and seafood are part of the program. You won't feel hungry on this program and you will be burning fat throughout the entire day. Success on this program depends on eating breakfast every day. If you do not eat breakfast, you will not succeed in loosing weight. It is as simple as that.

TAKING A LOOK AT KETOSIS

The key to the Atkins Diet and other high-protein, high-fat and low- or no-carbohydrate diets is ketosis. When you reduce your carbohydrate consumption considerably, your metabolism shifts and starts burning fat instead of glucose. After forty-eight hours with no carbohydrates, your insulin lowers, and your body shifts into ketosis. Triglycerides are broken down into ketone bodies. Ketosis is the state of burning fat. For those who want fast fat-burning results, ketosis provides this. Some people will lose three pounds a week by enhancing ketosis as recommended below.

How to Kick-Start Ketosis

If you want to kick start ketosis, eliminate all carbohydrates for forty-eight hours then revert to the regular Body Sense plan. Eat only healthy meats, wild fish, protein powders, free-range eggs (or tofu if you are vegetarian), low-glycemic (below 20) vegetables, and good fats from olive, flaxseed, and coconut. No fruits or fruit juices.

Ketones are by-products produced as a result of burning fat as fuel, which occurs during periods of low carbohydrate consumption. They are released in the urine and can be measured as an indicator of the state of ketosis or fat burning. Purchase ketone urine strips from the pharmacy so you can check daily to see if you are in ketosis. Follow the directions on the package. Once you have reached ketosis, your urine will test positive on the strip, and you will be burning fat. In a positive test, the stick will turn pink to a dark, reddish purple (the dark zone indicates extreme ketosis). Make sure you drink plenty of water, because concentrated urine due to dehydration can give false readings. You do not want to be in an extreme state of ketosis (the dark, reddish purple zone on the stick), as extreme ketosis creates a toxic substance (acetone0) that cannot be easily detoxi-fied by your body. When you have too much acetone in your body, your breath will smell terrible. The goal is not to be excessive, but to jump-start fat burning by staying in the low ketosis zone on the strips. Follow a healthy diet with an emphasis on protein, good fats, and low-glycemic index carbohydrates.

Is Ketosis Safe?

Ketogenic diets have been used for decades to control seizures in children with epilepsy. Research has also shown that the ketogenic diet is a useful tool in reducing tumor size in some cancers while ensuring adequate nutri-tion for the patient. Australian scientists found that diet-induced ketosis reduced melanoma, a deadly form of cancer. Several studies have evaluat-ed the safety of ketosis. In one study, morbidly obese (100 lbs/45 kg over their ideal weight) teenagers aged twelve to fifteen were placed on a keto-sis diet. Their average weight was 350 lbs (159 kg). After eight weeks on the ketogenic diet, they lost an average of 34 lbs (15.5 kg). The weight loss was exciting, but the big news is their blood chemistry remained normal throughout the study, and cholesterol levels dropped significantly. Obesity is rooted in too much insulin, and the ketogenic diet restores insulin to healthy levels.

Coconut Milk Stokes Ketosis

Medium-chain triglycerides (MCTs) can be found in coconut oil, and coconut milk. Coconut oil is the cheapest source and contains 50 percent MCTs. It can be heated for stir-fry and other sautéing. The Columbia Presbyterian Medical Center Children's hospital predominantly uses MCTs to induce ketosis in children who need this diet. Use coconut milk instead of the typical white flour or cornstarch in sauces—it is delicious and pro-motes weight loss.

Positive Results from Ketogenic Studies

Diets that promote ketosis have been extensively studied. Most people who are concerned about the safety of ketosis have heard about a serious side effect of diabetes called ketoacidosis. But the side effect is not the result of carbohydrate restriction; it is instead a side effect of uncontrolled diabetes. *Dr. Atkins' New Diet Revolution* coined a term called Benign Dietary Ketosis, which describes a beneficial fat-burning state caused by reducing carbohydrate, which causes the body to burn fat as fuel. There is much research using ketosis to treat disease and obesity.

Research shows ketosis:
- Lowers cholesterol in all studies to date
- Lowers triglycerides in all studies to date
- Balances blood sugar levels
- Normalizes uric acid levels, particularly useful for those with gout
- Promotes faster fat loss, especially in those needing to lose more than 30 pounds
- Supercharges fat burning, especially in teenagers who have been obese since childhood
- Relieves hypoglycemia by providing adequate fats and protein
- Promotes mental clarity, performance, and concentration, an effect felt after only a few days on the diet
- Inhibits cancer cell growth and is used in the clinical management of cancer
- Improves seizure control in children with epilepsy

Nothing is without side effects. The negative side of the ketogenic diet is bad breath, so chew parsley and drink real peppermint tea. Cravings for sugar can happen in the first few days. Stay busy by walking, shopping, or working. To reduce carbohydrate cravings, take 5-HTP, 50 to 100 mg three times per day. Constipation can also be a problem, so add 1 to 2 table-spoons of ground flaxseed to your food, eat more vegetables, and drink lots of water.

HYDRATE FOR FAT LOSS

We all know water is essential to life and to weight loss, but many people find it difficult to drink water. I found a way to make drinking water easy. I add unsweetened cranberry or other juices (pomegranate is wonderful), or I add herbal tea bags or slices of lemons or limes (after I have washed the skin) and grated fresh ginger, making the water more refreshing and palatable. Don't wait until you are thirsty to drink water, because you are dehydrated by then. Have up to eight glasses of water per day.

AVOID FAKE SWEETENERS

Synthetic sugar substitutes like aspartame (Nutrasweet™) and sucralose should be avoided. Aspartame is more sinful than sugar. It is a synthetic substance made up of phenylalanine, aspartic acid, and methanol (wood alcohol). Canada's Health Protection Branch regulates methanol, a potent neurotoxin, and has banned the food supplement phenylalanine for safety reasons, yet allows aspartame to be sold freely. Opponents of aspartame say there are links between aspartame and memory problems, seizure disorders, birth defects, headaches, and brain tumors. Although no long-term studies have proven these side effects, I recommend zylitol or stevia, two safe natural sweeteners.

A 1992 abstract published in *Science Health Abstracts* reported that sucralose, an artificial sweetener, shrank the thymus glands of rats up to 40 percent when taken in large doses. Because the thymus is so important to a healthy immune system, the Center for Science in the Public Interest requested that further studies be performed before sucralose was released in the United States. This request was ignored, and sucralose, sold under the name Splenda™, is available as a sweetener in North America today. Sucralose is a chlorinated sucrose derivative, with no long-term human research. Hundreds of animal studies have been performed using sucralose, some of which show hazards. Critics say the studies were inadequate.

NATURAL SWEETENERS

Stevia is a great alternative to artificial sweeteners. It is 300 times sweeter than sugar, has no calories, and is safe for diabetics. Stevia leaves have been used as herbal teas by diabetic patients in Asian countries. In a study published in 1993, no side effects were noted in diabetics who ate stevia for years. Two other research studies, published in 1981 and 1986, found that stevia extract can improve blood sugar levels.

Brazilian researchers at the Universities of São Paolo evaluated the role of stevia in blood sugar. Sixteen healthy volunteers were given extracts of

17 oz (5 g) of stevia leaves every six hours for three days. A glucose-tolerance test was performed before and after taking stevia, and the results were compared to another group who did not receive the stevia extracts. The study participants taking stevia had significantly lower blood sugar levels.

The sweet secret of stevia lies in a complex molecule called stevioside, which is a glycoside composed of glucose, sophorose, and steviol. It is this complex molecule and a number of other related compounds that account for the extraordinary sweetness of *Stevia rebaudiana*. Stevia is available in powder form for cooking and baking, and drops and tablets for coffee and tea.

Xylitol, another natural sweetener, was discovered in 1891 by German chemist Emil Fischer. It is a white crystalline powder, naturally occurring in fruits and vegetables. Xylitol has one-third fewer calories than white sugar. Xylitol reduces the development of dental cavities. Both stevia and xylitol are available in health food stores.

LEMON FOR DIGESTION

Each day you will start the morning with fresh-squeezed lemon juice (not lemon juice from a plastic bottle, but the real thing) or organic apple cider vinegar (white vinegar is often nothing more than a solution of acetic acid in water) in water; this helps flush and decongest the liver and stimulate digestion. You can use hot water, or squeeze lemon juice into your favorite herbal tea, especially ginger tea, which also aids fat loss. Lemon and water stimulate bile and promote the movement of wastes through the colon, speeding up elimination.

SLOWING GLUCOSE ABSORPTION

According to David Mendosa, most people know that when they eat protein, fat, or fiber, their blood glucose levels don't go up. Yet few of us are aware that there are foods that will *reduce* blood glucose. In one study, the glucose response when vinegar was eaten was 31 percent lower than without it. In another study vinegar significantly reduced the glycemic index of a starchy meal from 100 to 64. This is why you should start the day with fresh-squeezed lemon juice or apple cider vinegar in water or herbal tea, and use salad dressings made with organic apple cider or balsamic vinegars, essential fatty acid rich oils, and lemon juice. Mediterraneans dip their bread into olive oil and balsamic vinegar instead of slathering it with butter or margarine, thereby slowing the absorption of the glucose found in the bread and making it less fattening. Fermented foods like lactic acid-fermented sauerkraut, yogurt, fermented soy powders, and lactic acid-fermented pickles also reduce blood glucose levels.

FIBER FIGHTS FAT

Fiber from ground flaxseed provides lignans, which help your body eliminate excess estrogens and other toxins. Lignans are found predominantly in plants and can also be formed by bacteria in the gut. They have potent antiviral, antibacterial, and antifungal properties. Flaxseed is nature's most abundant source of lignans, with concentrations 75 to 800 times that of most other plant foods. Lignans bind to excess estrogens and eliminate potential cancer-causing estrogens, ensuring proper estrogen metabolism. Most of the research on flax has been done in Canada, the world supplier of flax. Researchers at the University of Toronto, Princess Margaret Hospital, and Toronto Hospital have shown that women with breast cancer who received 1 oz (25 g) of flaxseed daily experienced slower tumor growth. Researchers believe that adding flaxseed to the daily diet can prevent and treat breast cancer.

But we are talking about fat loss, you say. Even without lignans' benefits in reducing excess estrogens that can cause weight gain in both men and women, flaxseed is an excellent form of fiber, binding to estrogens and fat, bulking up the stool, and promoting mucilage to speed elimination. Take 2 tsps (10 mL) of ground flaxseed and mix it into a glass of water, then let it sit for a while. It will turn gelatinous and slippery (mucilage), which promotes effortless elimination. Flaxseed is an excellent source of omega-3 essential fatty acids, which research has shown to aid fat loss. Ground flaxseed is part of the Body Sense Natural Diet program. It ensures proper bowel movements, detoxification of excess estrogens, and binding of fat.

Lignans are also found in abundance in cranberries. Cranberries are important to any fat-burning program as they help mobilize fat from your cells and maintain a healthy liver. I recommend you add 1/2 cup (125 mL) of unsweetened cranberry juice to your big bottle of water to make it more palatable and to promote healthy fat metabolism in your liver. Cranberry juice, although it contains potent plant nutrients, does not contain lignans,

Flax Pudding	
This pudding tastes so good your family won't believe it is healthy.	
6 tbsps flaxseeds	90 mL
2 cups milk, soy milk, or Rice Dream™	500 mL
2 tbsps ground hazelnuts, almonds, or pistachios	30 mL
1 large banana, mashed	1
1 tbsp honey (optional)	15 mL
juice of one orange	
1 apple, peeled, cored, and grated	1
1 tbsp whipped cream (optional)	15 ml
strawberries or fresh fruit for garnish	

Pulse the flaxseeds in a coffee grinder for a few seconds. Bring milk to a boil in a double boiler. Add all the ground flaxseed at once and stir in with a whisk to prevent lumps. Boil for thirty seconds, remove from heat, and pour into a bowl. Let cool. It will have the consistency of pudding. Mix ground nuts, banana, honey, and orange juice into the flax pudding mixture. Gently mix in grated apple and spoon into parfait dishes, layered alternately with fresh fruit and real whipped cream. Top with a strawberry and a dab of whipped cream.

but the whole cranberry does. In addition to adding unsweetened cranberry juice to your water, take a cranberry capsule, an extremely potent form of cranberry. It takes 34 lbs (15.5 kg) of cranberries to produce 1 lb (.5 kg) of whole cranberry in capsules. Be sure to select a cranberry capsule in which all the vital parts of the berry are used, including the fruit, seeds, skin, and juice. Most cranberry capsule products use only dehydrated juice, which does not provide the benefits of the whole fruit.

SUPPLEMENTS TO SUPPORT FAT BURNING

Many nutritional supplements can support fat burning. Fats from flaxseed oil, evening primrose, and Conjugated Linoleic Acid (CLA), along with certain supplements, including Phase 2, curcumin, cayenne, green tea extract, milk thistle, rosemary, ginger, bitter orange, indole-3-carbinol, D-glucarate, sulforaphane, and protein powders, raise metabolism while improving liver function and facilitating hormone function for proper fat detoxification and elimination. See Chapter 6 for information on those supplements that support fat burning. If you have any health issues, you may need to add some food supplements to the Body Sense Natural Diet program. A multivitamin with minerals, protein powder, and digestive aids are required components of this program. I have yet to meet anyone who eats seven to ten half-cup (125 mL) servings of vegetables per day, which is the amount needed just to get basic vitamins and minerals. Protein powders raise metabolism and are a quick, easy way to get more protein into your diet. If you are older than thirty-five, have been dieting for years, or have eaten packaged foods over your lifetime, you need digestive enzymes or bitters, so those, too, are essential to success in this program.

LET'S GET STARTED!

You want results fast, and this program is designed to provide them. You have purchased the required foods and supplements, cleared your cupboards of harmful processed foods, and you are ready to get healthy. Fill out your daily journal (more on that in Chapter 3) and make sure you write down how you feel. After two weeks, measure your waist to see those inches falling off. Most diets ask you to visit your doctor's office to ensure that you are in perfect health. I have always thought this ironic. You are overweight, which means you are at risk for heart disease, diabetes, and certain cancers. In other words, you are not healthy. Along with the excess weight, you have no energy and may not have exercised in a while. If your doctor confirms all this, does that mean you can't diet? The Body Sense Natural Diet program is a new way of living—one that is simple to follow, safe, and successful.

Weight-Loss Tips

- Don't forget to take those pictures. You will want to show everyone when you are finished how different you look.
- Limit coffee to 1 cup (250 mL) (preferably organic) per day. Drink green tea the rest of the day; it is an excellent fat-attacking drink.
- Take your multivitamins with minerals every morning with breakfast.
- Eat protein for breakfast. Remember, it revs up your fat-burning furnace by 25 percent, and it stays revved up for six to eight hours. You can add protein powders to yogurt, cooked oatmeal, and other foods.
- Eat when you are hungry, but remember to choose healthy foods to snack on.

- Do not wait more than four hours between meals.
- Eat your food on a side plate; the dinner plate is too large, and you end up eating more than you need. Be reasonable about portion size, but don't measure and weigh the food. This program is for life, not just for six weeks.
- Use a big salad bowl and fill it with low-glycemic index vegetables and salad greens. You don't need to worry about portion size if you eat on a side plate and use a bowl for the veggies and salad.
- Put cayenne pepper in your pepper shaker instead of black pepper. Cayenne increases your fat-burning furnace.
- Use lemon juice and balsamic or apple cider vinegar on carbohydrates (vegetables, lentils, beans, pasta and breads) to slow the release of glucose.
- Chew your food well. Do not swallow until the food is thoroughly chewed.
- Drink water throughout the day. Try not to drink too many fluids with your meal, as this can dilute digestive juices and stomach acid.
- Take digestive enzymes with every meal and snack if you have been experiencing gas, bloating, burping, constipation, or have a distended abdomen.
- When sautéing vegetables, use coconut oil, extra virgin olive oil, or sesame oil sparingly. Water can be added, 1 tbsp (15 mL) at a time, to cut down on the amount of oil used.

GENERAL MEAL SUGGESTIONS

Keep these guidelines in mind when creating meals for your plan. I've provided 42 days of menus, but you can substitute your own creations using these helpful reminders on how to eat healthy.

- Dark green veggies such as broccoli, Brussels sprouts, asparagus, kale, romaine lettuce, mixed salad greens, spinach, arugula, and celery, etc. can be eaten without limit to serving size.
- Make sure you eat protein—chicken, eggs (scrambled, poached, soft or hard boiled, or omelette), protein powder, beef, fish, seafood, lentils, or tofu—at every meal.
- If you don't like plain water, add unsweetened cranberry juice to the water to give it flavor and/or drink naturally carbonated water with lime

or lemon. Use fresh-squeezed lemons or limes in the water, or add grated ginger. Water is essential to fat burning.

- During the first two weeks, no white foods are allowed. Thereafter, limit your intake of white foods (white pasta, white bread, white sugar, white flour, white rice). Remember, we call these the obesity foods.
- Use plain yogurt and add your own fruit to avoid artificial sweeteners and processed flavorings. Add protein powder to yogurt for a protein-enhanced snack.
- The only sweeteners allowed are stevia and xylitol, available at your health food store.
- Now that you aren't putting everything on bread, you can use vegetables as the foundation. Put smoked salmon or tuna between cucumber slices; use endive lettuce to hold nuts and bits of cheese; eat celery with salsa or fresh nut butters; wrap cheese around your burger; use mounds of sprouts, instead of rice or pasta, to hold sauces and veggies; a hard-boiled egg without the yolk can hold foods; an avocado is a great cup for holding crabmeat, tuna, and chopped herbs.

Let's look at breakfast, lunch, dinner, and snacks to see how we can make the tastiest and most effective food decisions while following this plan.

Breakfast

The most important meal of the day can be varied and delicious even when you're on a diet. Check out these yummy suggestions that are easy to prepare.

Smoothies of all types are a great breakfast and snack food. Experiment with protein powders until you find one that you enjoy eating.

Eggs can be used in hundreds of creative ways: quiches without the crust, soft-boiled eggs, omelettes, frittatas with cheese and veggies. Use super-thin omelettes like crêpes and fill with meats, vegetables, and sprouts.

Cook extra chicken breasts and put them in an airtight container to eat cold with a little salt or yogurt with dill dressing in the morning. Salmon lox can be rolled around veggies and hard-boiled eggs. Lox can also be used in place of toast with poached eggs.

Make large-cut, old-fashioned oatmeal (not the instant type) and, once cooked, add two scoops of plain or vanilla protein powder to have all the benefits of protein with your cooked cereal. Add some peaches and enjoy.

Lunch and Dinner

The main meals of your day can be delicious. No need to eat the same foods day after day. With my plan you can enjoy a wonderful variety of lunches and dinners.

- Homemade soups can last a couple of days and provide a quick meal. I make huge batches and freeze individual servings in yogurt containers. Or purchase good-quality soups—black bean, lentil, or meat-based—without added sugar (read the label for glucose, fructose, or other sweeteners). Stock the cupboards with these.
- Broiled or baked chicken marinated in lemon, accompanied by a salad, makes a good meal.
- Hamburger patties can be eaten with lettuce, tomato, cheese, and onion toppings. If you must eat at a fast-food restaurant, order your burger without the bun. Always say no to the bread.
- Canned tuna, crabmeat, wild salmon, sardines, and oysters are quick, easy ways to get instant protein.
- Cook chili with meat and beans (if buying canned, ensure that it has no glucose, fructose, or flour). Freeze leftovers for later use.
- Vegetables can be eaten raw or cooked. Wash and bag veggies for the week. You will eat more veggies if they are ready to eat.

Snacks

Consider these tasty treats when you need something to snack on.

- organic nuts—no more than twenty per day
- low-carb, protein-enriched bars
- hard-boiled eggs
- protein powders
- veggies with hummus
- fruits below 20 on the glycemic index list, only one per day

Dessert

Think dieting means no dessert? Not so! See the delectable options below.

- flax pudding (see recipe earlier in this chapter)
- cottage cheese with fruit
- banana dipped in real whipped cream (no sugar added)
- plain yogurt with chocolate protein powder (this tastes like cheesecake)
- meal replacement: mix and let stand in the refrigerator until cold. It makes a nice pudding.

THE DIET PLAN

This plan couldn't be easier to follow. Imagine—no measuring! I have not provided serving sizes for each meal plan, because when you eat foods low on the glycemic index (below 60) and you follow the 10-minute exercise program, you do not have to be too concerned about measuring every portion. When it comes to pasta or bread, serving sizes must be strictly adhered to, but I want you to learn how to eat for the long term, and you are probably too busy to spend every day measuring and weighing your food. Remember, you can eat as many greens and green vegetables as you like. Your protein portions—meat, chicken, egg, fish, seafood, and tofu—can be large as long as you are not covering them with sauces that are not acceptable.

For the first three days, you will eat mainly protein—including chicken, cheese, protein powders, lean red meat, eggs, fish, or tofu—and healthy fats until you are in ketosis. Vegetarians often do not get enough protein, even those who are very careful about food combining. It is imperative if you are a vegetarian that you eat tofu, beans, legumes, nuts, and seeds or, if you are lacto-ovo vegetarian, that you eat eggs or cheese as alternatives to the animal-based protein recommended in the following diet. Eating protein is a major component in the success of this program.

Day One

Upon rising, drink 8 oz (250 mL) hot water or herbal tea with fresh-squeezed lemon juice.

Breakfast
- Veggie scramble: two eggs with asparagus or broccoli, onions, or peppers; use coconut butter in the sauté pan
- Green tea or coffee; sweeten with stevia and add milk or cream as desired

Snack
- Half a small chicken breast or a piece of cheese
- Green tea

Lunch
- Green salad with lemon juice or balsamic vinegar and extra-virgin olive oil
- Half a can of drained, water-packed tuna

Snack
- Protein powder shake mixed into water, nut or rice milk (as directed on the label of the protein powder)

Dinner
- Baked fish
- Green salad with olive oil or flaxseed oil

Day Two

Upon rising, drink 8 oz (250 mL) hot water or herbal tea with fresh-squeezed lemon juice.

Breakfast
- Protein powder smoothie (place ice, protein powder, and one cup/250 mL unsweetened yogurt in to blender and blend until smooth)
- Green tea or coffee; sweeten with stevia and add milk or cream as desired

Snack
- Hard-boiled egg
- Green tea

Lunch
- Veggies and half a small grilled chicken breast

Snack
- One 2-inch (5-cm) piece of hard cheese (not processed slices)

Dinner
- Flank steak, grilled or roasted with garlic
- Dark green vegetable of your choice
- Green salad with extra-virgin olive oil/balsamic vinegar

Day Three

Upon rising, drink 8 oz (250 mL) hot water or herbal tea with fresh-squeezed lemon juice.

Breakfast
- 1/2 cup (125 mL) plain organic yogurt with two scoops of vanilla protein powder; sprinkle with cinnamon or cardamom
- Green tea or coffee; sweeten with stevia and add milk or cream as desired

Snack
- Twelve almonds or other nuts

Lunch
- Baked turkey breast with green veggies or salad

Snack
- Hard-boiled egg

Dinner
- Tofu stir-fry with broccoli, onions, and garlic

*Now you should be in the accelerated fat burning mode (ketosis) —check the Ketostix to be sure, and if you are, you can add more green vegetables and the good carbohydrates (those rated below 60 on the glycemic index) to your meals.

Day Four

Upon rising, drink 8 oz (250 mL) of hot water or herbal tea with fresh-squeezed lemon juice.

Breakfast
- Egg, soft or hard boiled, scrambled, or poached
- One slice of whole-grain rye or pumpernickel bread with better butter (see recipe earlier in this chapter)
- Green tea or coffee; sweeten with stevia and add milk or cream as desired

Snack
- Protein powder shake
- Glass of water

Lunch
- Grilled chicken breast without the skin
- Green salad with ginger dressing
- Glass of water

Snack
- Ten large cherries or one nectarine
- Green tea

Dinner
- Broiled steak, burger, or tofu burger
- Dark green veggies
- Coleslaw with extra-virgin olive oil and vinegar
- Glass of water

Day Five

Upon rising, drink 8 oz (250 mL) hot water or herbal tea with fresh-squeezed lemon juice.

Breakfast
- 1 cup (250 mL) plain yogurt, with 1 tbsp (15 mL) ground flaxseed (available from a health food store or grind your own seeds in a small coffee grinder) and two scoops of protein powder
- Green tea or coffee; sweeten with stevia and add milk or cream as desired

Snack
- Two plums or half a pink grapefruit

Lunch
- 1 cup (250 mL) lentil or vegetable soup (if using canned soup, ensure that it does not contain any sugar, glucose, or fructose)
- Hard-boiled egg
- Glass of water

Snack
- Protein powder shake with banana
- Glass of water

Dinner
- 1/2 cup (125 mL) whole-grain pasta with 1 cup (250 mL) tomato sauce with ground turkey
- Green vegetable side salad with flaxseed oil, crushed garlic, and lemon
- Glass of water

Day Six

Upon rising, drink 8 oz (250 mL) hot water or herbal tea with fresh-squeezed lemon juice.

Breakfast
- 1 cup/ 250 mL of blueberries and plain yogurt mixed with 2 scoops of protein powder
- Green tea or coffee; sweeten with stevia and add milk or cream as desired

Snack
- Low-carb protein bar
- Glass of water

Lunch
- Omelette with peppers, onions, mushroom, 2 tbsps (30 mL) real cheddar or Monterey Jack cheese, and 1 tbsp (15 mL) salsa
- Green salad with extra-virgin olive oil, lemon juice, and cayenne pepper
- Glass of water

Snack
- One peach or 1/2 cup (125 mL) canned unsweetened peaches

Dinner
- 4 oz (115 g) shrimp with garlic, onions, fresh sugar snap peas, or baby corn

- Endive, radicchio, and arugula salad with yogurt, herb, lemon, cayenne, and flaxseed oil dressing
- Glass of water

Day Seven

Upon rising, drink 8 oz (250 mL) hot water or herbal tea with fresh-squeezed lemon juice.

Breakfast
- One slice of whole-grain rye or pumpernickel bread
- Two eggs, poached, boiled, or scrambled
- Green tea or coffee; sweeten with stevia and add milk or cream as desired

Snack
- Protein powder shake with one small banana
- Glass of water

Lunch
- Turkey, all-beef, or tofu burger without the bun; ensure condiments (mustard, relish, ketchup) do not contain sugar
- Vegetable salad

Snack
- One peach

Dinner
- Spicy Thai dinner with chicken or beef
- Sautéed vegetables with tamari or soy sauce and freshly grated ginger

Day 8

Upon rising, drink 8 oz (250 mL) hot water or herbal tea with fresh-squeezed lemon juice.

Breakfast
- Smoked salmon wrapped around a hard-boiled egg or asparagus spears
- Green tea or coffee; sweeten with stevia and add milk or cream as desired

Snack
- 1 (2 oz) mozzarella cheese stick

Lunch
- 1/2 grilled chicken breast
- Mixed green salad with garlic, chili, and flaxseed oil

Snack
- 1/2 cup (125 mL) cottage cheese with berries

Dinner
- Cornish game hen, roasted
- 1/2 cup (125 mL) yams
- Green vegetables

Day 9

Upon rising, drink 8 oz (250 mL) hot water or herbal tea with fresh-squeezed lemon juice.

Breakfast
- Broccoli and scallions sautéed with 2 scrambled eggs (for ease, make this all in the same pan)
- Green tea or coffee; sweeten with stevia and add milk or cream as desired

Snack
- Raw vegetables with sour cream and herb dip

Lunch
- Half an avocado stuffed with crab meat and chopped green onions

Snack
- Protein smoothie with banana

Dinner
- 1/2 cup (125 mL) egg fettuccine with 1/2 cup (125 mL) tofu or cooked ground turkey crumbled into spaghetti sauce
- Green salad dressed with extra virgin olive oil mixed with balsamic vinegar and herbs

Day 10

Upon rising, drink 8 oz (250 mL) hot water or herbal tea with fresh-squeezed lemon juice.

Breakfast
- 2 poached eggs on one slice of dark rye toast spread with 1/2 tsp (2.5 mL) better butter
- Green tea or coffee; sweeten with stevia and add milk or cream as desired

Snack
- 1/2 cup (125 mL) yogurt with 1/3 cup (75 mL) berries

Lunch
- 1 cup (250 mL) black bean soup
- Veggies and dip

Snack
- Celery stuffed with hummus or cream cheese

Dinner
- Poached salmon topped with 4 tbsp (50 mL) yogurt mixed with chopped dill
- Green salad with salad dressing made of hemp seed oil, garlic, and yogurt (mix to taste)

Day 11

Upon rising, drink 8 oz (250 mL) hot water or herbal tea with fresh-squeezed lemon juice.

Breakfast
- 1/2 cup (125 mL) cooked oatmeal with 2 scoops vanilla protein powder and 1/2 cup (125 mL) unsweetened rice or nut milk

- Green tea or coffee; sweeten with stevia and add milk or cream as desired

Snack

- 1/2 cup (150 mL) blueberries

Lunch

- Turkey roll-up: wrap turkey slices around lettuce and grated carrots, then spread turkey with 1/2 tsp (2.5 mL) mayonnaise

Snack

- Protein shake

Dinner

- Halibut baked with lemon and capers
- Green vegetables of your choice
- 1/2 small yam, baked with 1 tsp (5 mL) better butter

Day 12

Upon rising, drink 8 oz (250 mL) hot water or herbal tea with fresh-squeezed lemon juice.

Breakfast

- 2 scoops of protein powder mixed into 1/2 cup (125 mL) plain yogurt with 1 tbsp (15 mL) ground flaxseeds
- Green tea or coffee; sweeten with stevia and add milk or cream as desired

Snack

- 1 small peach or pear or 1/2 cup (125 mL) canned, unsweetened peaches or pears

Lunch

- 1/2 cup (125 mL) cottage cheese with raw vegetables

Snack

- Cucumber slices with Havarti or Swiss cheese on top

Dinner

- Curry vegetables and tofu (or chicken)
- Mixed green salad with extra virgin olive oil, garlic, yogurt, and chives

Day 13

Upon rising, drink 8 oz (250 mL) hot water or herbal tea with fresh-squeezed lemon juice.

Breakfast

- 1 hard-boiled egg mashed with 1 tbsp (15 mL) mayonnaise, spread over lettuce pieces
- Green tea or coffee; sweeten with stevia and add milk or cream as desired

Snack

- 12 almonds or macadamia nuts
- Glass of water

Lunch

- Meal replacement shake (see Appendix)
- Mixed green salad and chopped veggies with extra virgin olive oil and lemon juice

Snack
- 1/2 can tuna dressed with 1 tbsp (15 mL) real egg mayonnaise

Dinner
- Lean steak broiled with garlic and cracked peppercorns
- 1/2 small yam
- Green vegetables

Day 14

Upon rising, drink 8 oz (250 mL) hot water or herbal tea with fresh-squeezed lemon juice.

Breakfast
- 1/2 cup (125 mL) cooked oatmeal, with 2 scoops protein powder and 1/2 cup (125 mL) unsweetened rice or nut milk
- Green tea or coffee; sweeten with stevia and add milk or cream as desired

Snack
- 1 cup (250 mL) cherries
- 1–2 tbsp (15–30 mL) sunflower seeds or raw nuts

Lunch
- Salmon burger or tofu burger wrapped in several layers of lettuce, with tomato and onion slices; (make sure condiments contain no sugar, glucose, or fructose)

Snack
- Raw veggies and sour cream dip

Dinner
- 1 cup (250 mL) of real egg fettuccini with creamy Alfredo sauce (optional: add grilled chicken)
- Green vegetables of your choice

Day 15

Upon rising, drink 8 oz (250 mL) hot water or herbal tea with fresh-squeezed lemon juice.

Breakfast
- Two-egg omelet filled with sautéed broccoli, asparagus spears, and peppers
- Green tea or coffee; sweeten with stevia and add milk or cream as desired

Snack
- 1 cup (250 mL) mixed fruit (fresh, or canned unsweetened)

Lunch
- Meal replacement shake (see Appendix)
- Glass of water

Snack
- 1 piece of cheese and 12 almonds

Dinner
- Ground turkey tacos with grated cheese, sour cream, salsa, chopped tomatoes, and avocado
- Mixed green salad dressed with olive oil, balsamic vinegar, and herbs

Day 16

Upon rising, drink 8 oz (250 mL) hot water or herbal tea with fresh-squeezed lemon juice.

Breakfast
- Pancakes made from low-carb mix, available from the health food store or specialty section of your grocery store. Top with 1/2 cup (125 mL) mixed unsweetened canned or fresh fruit and 1/4 cup (62.5 mL) unsweetened whipped cream.
- Green tea or coffee; sweeten with stevia and add milk or cream as desired

Snack
- Protein shake

Lunch
- Salad with turkey slices, grated cheese, olives, artichoke hearts, and creamy dressing

Snack
- 12 nuts and/or 2 oz of cheese
- 1 glass of water

Dinner
- Pork tenderloin slices stir-fried with carrots, peppers, baby corn, mung bean sprouts, ginger, garlic, and soy sauce

Day 17

Upon rising, drink 8 oz (250 ml) hot water or herbal tea with fresh-squeezed lemon juice.

Breakfast
- 2 eggs any style with one slice of dark rye toast and 1/2 tsp(2.5 mL) better butter
- Green tea or coffee; sweeten with stevia and add milk or cream as desired

Snack
- Protein smoothie with 1/4 cup (62.5 mL) cranberries and 1/2 banana

Lunch
- Vegetable beef soup
- Mixed green salad dressed with creamy dressing

Snack
- Raw vegetables with hummus dip

Dinner
- Grilled skewered chicken marinated in garlic, oregano, and lemon
- Mixed green salad with black olives and marinated artichoke hearts dressed with extra virgin olive oil, garlic, and lemon

Day 18

Upon rising, drink 8 oz (250 mL) hot water or herbal tea with fresh-squeezed lemon juice.

Breakfast
- Flaxseed pudding with 1/3 cup fresh fruit
- Green tea or coffee; sweeten with stevia and add milk or cream as desired

Snack
- Protein shake
- Glass of water

Lunch
- Ahi tuna salad drizzled with lime juice served over a bed of baby romaine lettuce

Snack
- Cheese and cucumber slices

Dinner
- Broiled steak with steamed green vegetables
- 1/2 small yam with 1 tbsp (15 mL) better butter

Day 19

Upon rising, drink 8 oz (250 mL) hot water or herbal tea with fresh-squeezed lemon juice.

Breakfast
- 1 poached egg served on a bed of steamed spinach with grated cheese
- Green tea or coffee; sweeten with stevia and add milk or cream as desired

Snack
- Celery stuffed with hummus, nut butter, or Brie cheese

Lunch
- Avocado stuffed with canned crab meat, chopped chives, and 1 tbsp (15 mL) real egg mayonnaise

Snack
- 1 peach or pear, fresh or 1/2 (125 mL) cup canned unsweetened

Dinner
- Hearty beef and bean chili with grated cheese
- Mixed green salad with raspberry dressing

Day 20

Upon rising, drink 8 oz (250 mL) hot water or herbal tea with fresh-squeezed lemon juice.

Breakfast
- 2 slices peameal or back bacon (Canadian bacon)
- 1 egg any style
- 1 slice of dark rye toast with 1 tbsp (15 mL) better butter or coconut butter
- Green tea or coffee; sweeten with stevia and add milk or cream as desired

Snack
• Red pepper slices spread with Brie or Camembert cheese or hummus
Lunch
• Salmon or veggie burger wrapped in several lettuce leaves garnished with tomato, cheese, onions, and sugar-free condiments
Snack
• Endive lettuce filled with tuna or canned crabmeat garnished with chopped green onions
Dinner
• Low-carb tortilla wrap filled with chopped grilled chicken breast, onions, peppers, celery topped with cheese and salsa
• Mixed green salad with creamy dressing

Day 21
Upon rising, drink 8 oz (250 mL) hot water or herbal tea with fresh-squeezed lemon juice.
Breakfast
• Smoked salmon or lox on rye crisp spread with cream cheese and topped with capers
• Green tea or coffee; sweeten with stevia and add milk or cream as desired
Snack
• Hard-boiled egg
Lunch
• Hearty lentil or chicken vegetable soup
• 1 slice of low carb bread with 1 tbsp (15 mL) better butter
Snack
• 1 pear, peach, or banana
Dinner
• Baked chicken breast in curry sauce (curry sauces come in many flavors and are available in jars at the grocery store; buy one that does not contain sugar, glucose, or fructose)
• Cauliflower
• 1/2 small baked yam with 1 tsp (5 mL) better butter

Day 22
Upon rising, drink 8 oz (250 mL) hot water or herbal tea with fresh-squeezed lemon juice.
Breakfast
• Pancakes made from low-carb mix available from the health food store or specialty section of your grocery store; top with 1/2 cup (125 mL) cup mixed unsweetened canned or fresh fruit and 1/4 cup (62.5 mL) unsweetened whipped cream
• Green tea or coffee; sweeten with stevia and add milk or cream as desired

Snack
- 1 hard-boiled egg

Lunch
- Vegetable stir-fry with chicken, beef, or tofu
- 1/2 cup (125 mL) cup brown or wild rice

Snack
- 2 oz (50 g) of mozzarella cheese

Dinner
- Roast beef
- Oven-roasted vegetables
- 1/2 small yam with 1 tsp (5 mL) better butter

Day 23

Upon rising drink 8 oz (250 mL) hot water or herbal tea with fresh-squeezed lemon juice.

Breakfast
- 1/2 cup (125 mL) plain organic yogurt with 2 scoops of protein powder, with 1/4 cup (62.5) berries
- Green tea or coffee; sweeten with stevia and add milk or cream as desired

Snack
- Celery stuffed with nut butter, hummus, or Brie cheese

Lunch
- Turkey, chicken, or roast beef slices; spread 1 tbsp (15 mL) real egg mayonnaise or unsweetened mustard on meat, then wrap meat around grated carrots and lettuce

Snack
- 12 almonds or 2 tbsp (30 mL) soy nuts
- Glass of water

Dinner
- 1 cup (250 mL) real egg fettuccini with primavera sauce (vegetables in tomato sauce); add pitted Kalamata olives and dust with grated Parmesan cheese
- Mixed green salad with olive oil, balsamic vinegar, and herbs

Day 24

Upon rising, drink 8 oz (250 mL) hot water or herbal tea with fresh-squeezed lemon juice.

Breakfast
- 1/2 cup (125 mL) cooked oatmeal with 2 scoops of vanilla protein powder and 1/2 cup (125 mL) of rice or nut milk
- Green tea or coffee; sweeten with stevia and add milk or cream as desired

Snack
- Turkey slices wrapped around cheese

Lunch
- Lentil, black bean, chicken, or beef with vegetable soup
- Mixed green salad with creamy dressing

Snack
- 1 hard-boiled egg

Dinner
- Flank steak marinated in garlic and soy sauce then baked and sliced thinly
- Green vegetables

Day 25

Upon rising, drink 8 oz (250 mL) hot water or herbal tea with fresh-squeezed lemon juice.

Breakfast
- 1 egg any style
- 2 slices of peameal or back bacon (Canadian bacon)
- Green tea or coffee; sweeten with stevia and add milk or cream as desired

Snack
- Endive lettuce stuffed with walnuts and crumbled feta or blue cheese

Lunch
- Niçoise salad with tuna, chopped egg, green beans, olives, peppers, mixed greens, and olive oil and wine vinaigrette

Snack
- Protein shake

Dinner
- Stir-fried shrimp and vegetables with garlic, ginger, and olive oil
- 1/2 cup (125 mL) brown or wild rice

Day 26

Upon rising, drink 8 oz (250 mL) hot water or herbal tea with fresh-squeezed lemon juice.

Breakfast
- 2 poached eggs on smoked salmon, grilled sausage patty, or back bacon
- Green tea or coffee; sweeten with stevia and add milk or cream as desired

Snack
- 1/2 cup (125 mL) cottage cheese with berries

Lunch
- Turkey or chicken slices spread with 1 tbsp (15 mL) real egg mayonnaise or mustard; wrap the meat around red pepper sticks, asparagus spears, or cheese.

Snack
- 1 small mango

Dinner
- Turkey breast, sautéed with rosemary and thyme
- Spaghetti squash, baked
- Brussels sprouts
- Caesar salad (no croutons)

Day 27

Upon rising, drink 8 oz (250 mL) hot water or herbal tea with fresh-squeezed lemon juice.
Breakfast
- 1/2 cup (125 mL) cooked oatmeal with 2 scoops of vanilla protein powder with 1/2 cup (125 mL) of rice or nut milk
- Green tea or coffee; sweeten with stevia and add milk or cream as desired
Snack
- 2 large pieces of watermelon or cantaloupe
Lunch
- Omelette with peppers, onions, mushroom, 2 tbsp (30 mL) real cheddar or Monterey Jack cheese, and 1 tbsp (15 mL) salsa
- Green salad with extra-virgin olive oil, lemon, and cayenne pepper
- Glass of water
Snack
- Red pepper slices spread with Brie or Camembert cheese or hummus
Dinner
- Pork tenderloin slices stir-fried with carrots, peppers, baby corn, mung bean sprouts, ginger, garlic, and soy sauce

Day 28

Upon rising, drink 8 oz (250 mL) hot water or herbal tea with fresh-squeezed lemon juice.
Breakfast
- Veggie scramble: two eggs with asparagus or broccoli, onions, or peppers; use coconut butter in the sauté pan; it is an excellent source of medium-chain triglycerides to enhance thyroid and improve metabolism
- Green tea or coffee; sweeten with stevia and add milk or cream as desired
Snack
- Protein powder smoothie (place ice, protein powder and 1/2 cup (125 mL) unsweetened yogurt into blender and blend until smooth)
Lunch
- Shrimp, chicken, or tofu grilled and served on a bed of mixed greens
- Lemon, herb, and olive oil dressing
Snack
- 1 nectarine

Dinner
- Hearty beef and bean chili with grated cheese
- Mixed green salad with creamy dressing

Day 29

Upon rising, drink 8 oz (250 mL) hot water or herbal tea with fresh-squeezed lemon juice.
Breakfast
- Mushroom and cheese omelette
- Green tea or coffee; sweeten with stevia and add milk or cream as desired

Snack
- Protein smoothie with blueberries

Lunch
- Grilled turkey burger or veggie burger
- Greek salad with chopped tomatoes, cucumber, onions, feta cheese, and olives; dress with extra virgin olive oil, balsamic vinegar, and crushed garlic

Snack
- 1/2 cup (125 mL) cottage cheese with raw vegetables

Dinner
- 1 cup (250 mL) real egg fettuccini with primavera sauce (broccoli, onions, peppers, celery, and capers in tomato sauce) dusted with grated Parmesan cheese
- Mixed green salad with olive oil, balsamic vinegar, and herbs

Day 30

Upon rising, drink 8 oz (250 mL) hot water or herbal tea with fresh-squeezed lemon juice.
Breakfast
- Smoked salmon or lox on rye crisp spread with cream cheese; top with capers
- Green tea or coffee; sweeten with stevia and add milk or cream as desired

Snack
- Celery with nut butter, hummus

Lunch
- 1/2 can of tuna or wild salmon served on a bed of baby greens with creamy dressing

Snack
- 1 peach or pear (fresh) or 1/2 cup (125 mL) canned, unsweetened

Dinner
- Ground turkey tacos with grated cheese, sour cream, salsa, chopped tomatoes, and avocado
- Mixed green salad dressed with olive oil, balsamic vinegar, and herbs

Day 31

Upon rising, drink 8 oz (250 mL) hot water or herbal tea with fresh-squeezed lemon juice.

Breakfast
- 2 slices of peameal bacon (Canadian bacon)
- 1 egg any style
- 1 slice of dark rye toast with 1 tbsp (15 mL) better butter
- Green tea or coffee; sweeten with stevia and add milk or cream as desired

Snack
- Protein smoothie with strawberries

Lunch
- Rye crisp bread with Brie or Camembert cheese
- Mixed green salad with creamy dressing

Snack
- Cucumber or tomato with mozzarella cheese

Dinner
- Lean steak broiled with garlic, cracked peppercorns
- 1/2 small yam
- Green vegetables

Day 32

Upon rising, drink 8 oz (250 mL) hot water or herbal tea with fresh-squeezed lemon juice.

Breakfast
- 2 scrambled eggs with cilantro, tomatoes and chives
- Green tea or coffee; sweeten with stevia and add milk or cream as desired

Snack
- 1/2 cup (125 mL) plain yogurt with 2 scoops of chocolate protein powder

Lunch
- Spinach salad with tomatoes, feta, and almonds served with raspberry vinaigrette

Snack
- 1 hard-boiled egg

Dinner
- Baked chicken breast in curry sauce (available in jars at the grocery store; buy a sauce that does not contain sugar, glucose, or fructose)
- Cauliflower
- 1/2 small baked yam with 1 tsp (5 mL) of better butter

Day 33

Upon rising, drink 8 oz (250 mL) hot water or herbal tea with fresh-squeezed lemon juice.

Breakfast
• Turkey or black forest ham wrapped around 2 hard-boiled eggs
• Green tea or coffee; sweeten with stevia and add milk or cream as desired

Snack
• Protein powder smoothie (place ice, protein powder, and 1/2 cup (125 mL) unsweetened yogurt in blender and blend until smooth)

Lunch
• Spicy chicken wings or drum sticks
• Raw veggies with sour cream and chive dip

Snack
• 1 piece of cheese (2 oz)
• Glass of water

Dinner
• Stir-fried shrimp and vegetables with garlic, ginger, and olive oil
• 1/2 cup (125 mL) brown or wild rice

Day 34

Upon rising, drink 8 oz (250 mL) hot water or herbal tea with fresh-squeezed lemon juice.

Breakfast
• 1/2 cup (125 mL) cup cottage cheese with 1/2 cup (125 mL) cup mixed fruit
• Green tea or coffee; sweeten with stevia and add milk or cream as desired

Snack
• Protein shake

Lunch
• Shaved beef or lamb served on mixed lettuces with spicy dressing

Snack
• 1 nectarine

Dinner
• Grilled fish (tuna, halibut, or salmon)
• Green vegetables
• 1/2 cup (125 mL) brown or wild rice

Day 35

Upon rising, drink 8 oz (250 mL) hot water or herbal tea with fresh-squeezed lemon juice.

Breakfast
• Protein smoothie, peach
• Green tea or coffee; sweeten with stevia and add milk or cream as desired

Snack
- 1 hard-boiled egg

Lunch
- Rye crisp bread with nut butter or chicken, turkey, or ham (spread meat with 1 tsp (5 mL) real egg mayonnaise or unsweetened mustard)
- Mixed green salad with creamy dressing

Snack
- 12 almonds or other nuts

Dinner
- Grilled tuna or salmon steak with lemon and capers
- 1/2 small baked yam with 1 tsp (5 mL) better butter
- Green vegetables

Day 36

Upon rising, drink 8 oz (250 mL) hot water or herbal tea with fresh-squeezed lemon juice.

Breakfast
- 1/2 cup (125 mL) cup cooked oatmeal with 2 scoops of vanilla protein powder and 1/2 cup (125 mL) rice or nut milk
- Green tea or coffee; sweeten with stevia and add milk or cream as desired

Snack
- Low-carb protein bar

Lunch
- Hearty beef or chicken vegetable soup
- Mixed green salad with creamy dressing

Snack
- Banana dipped in real unsweetened whipped cream

Dinner
- 1/2 cup (125 mL) real egg fettuccine with spaghetti sauce and meat balls (ensure the meat balls are not filled with bread)
- Steamed green vegetables

Day 37

Upon rising, drink 8 oz (250 mL) hot water or herbal tea with fresh-squeezed lemon juice.

Breakfast
- Asparagus or broccoli two-egg omelette
- Green tea or coffee; sweeten with stevia and add milk or cream as desired

Snack
- 1/2 grapefruit

Lunch
- Stir-fried tofu, chicken, or shrimp and vegetable served over plenty of sautéed mung bean sprouts

Snack
- Protein smoothie with raspberries

Dinner
- Grilled lamb chop
- 1/2 small baked yam with 1 tsp (5 mL) better butter
- Steamed green beans with freshly grated ginger

Day 38

Upon rising, drink 8 oz (250 mL) hot water or herbal tea with fresh-squeezed lemon juice.

Breakfast
- Veggie scramble: two eggs with asparagus or broccoli, onions, or peppers
- Green tea or coffee; sweeten with stevia and add milk or cream as desired

Snack
- Protein powder smoothie (place ice, protein powder and 1/2 cup (125 mL) unsweetened yogurt in blender and blend until smooth)

Lunch
- Turkey, chicken, or ham slices spread with 1 tsp (5 mL) real egg mayonnaise or mustard; wrap the meat around cheese and red pepper or asparagus pieces

Snack
- 1/2 cup (125 mL) cup cherries

Dinner
- Pork tenderloin slices stir-fried with carrots, peppers, baby corn, ginger, garlic, and soy sauce served on a big bed of sautéed mung bean sprouts

Day 39

Upon rising, drink 8 oz (250 mL) hot water or herbal tea with fresh-squeezed lemon juice.

Breakfast
- Black Forest ham wrapped around a hard-boiled egg
- Green tea or coffee; sweeten with stevia and add milk or cream as desired

Snack
- Protein smoothie with 1/4 cup (62.5 mL) cup cranberries

Lunch
- Spicy chicken wings or drumsticks
- Raw veggies with sour cream and chive dip

Snack
- Celery stuffed with hummus, nut butter, or cheese

Dinner
- Sautéed ginger shrimp and snow peas served on 1/2 cup (125 mL) brown rice with tamari or soy sauce to taste

Day 40

Upon rising, drink 8 oz (250 mL) hot water or herbal tea with fresh-squeezed lemon juice.

Breakfast
- 2 slices of peameal bacon (Canadian bacon)
- 1 egg any style
- 1 slice of dark rye toast with 1 tsp (15 mL) of better butter
- Green tea or coffee; sweeten with stevia and add milk or cream as desired

Snack
- 1 nectarine or peach

Lunch
- One ground-turkey or ground-beef taco with grated cheese, sour cream, spicy salsa, chopped tomatoes, and avocado

Snack
- 1/2 cup (125 mL) cottage cheese
- Raw veggies

Dinner
- 1 cup (250 mL) real egg fettuccini with primavera sauce (vegetables in tomato sauce) and pitted Kalamata olives, dusted with grated Parmesan cheese
- Mixed green salad with olive oil, balsamic vinegar, and herbs

---

Day 41

Upon rising, drink 8 oz (250 mL) hot water or herbal tea with fresh-squeezed lemon juice.

Breakfast
- 1/2 cup (125 mL) cooked oatmeal with 2 scoops of vanilla protein powder and 1/2 cup (125 mL) rice or nut milk
- Green tea or coffee; sweeten with stevia and add milk or cream as desired

Snack
- Protein powder smoothie (place ice, protein powder and 1 cup (250 mL) of unsweetened yogurt in blender and blend until smooth)

Lunch
- Niçoise salad with tuna, chopped egg, green beans, olives, peppers, mixed greens with olive oil and wine vinaigrette

Snack
- 1 hard-boiled egg or a piece of cheese

Dinner
- Roast beef
- Oven-roasted vegetables
- 1/2 small yam with 1 tsp (5 mL) better butter

Day 42

Upon rising, drink 8 oz (250 mL) hot water or herbal tea with fresh-squeezed lemon juice.

Breakfast
- Pancakes made from low-carb mix, available from the health food store or specialty section of your grocery store. Top with 1/2 cup (125 mL) mixed unsweetened canned or fresh fruit and 1/4 cup (62.5 mL) unsweetened whipped cream.
- Green tea or coffee; sweeten with stevia and add milk or cream as desired

Snack
- Cucumber spread with nut butter, hummus, or cheese

Lunch
- Hearty beef or chicken vegetable soup
- Mixed green salad with creamy dressing

Snack
- Endive pieces filled with feta or blue cheese and walnuts

Dinner
- Skewered chicken marinated in garlic, oregano, and lemon, then grilled
- Mixed green salad with black olives and marinated artichoke hearts dressed with extra virgin olive oil, garlic, and lemon

---

I have provided six weeks of delicious menu ideas. Now you can proceed to make up your own meals. Always include protein and vegetables. Choose foods low on the glycemic index. You are on your way to losing weight and feeling fabulous. Remember to look in the mirror every day and tell yourself what a wonderful person you are and how great you look. Chapter 3 will help you understand the emotional side of eating, how to change food cravings, and how your personal brain biochemistry can work with you or against you as you set out to stay in shape.

chapter three

Emotional Eating

Scientists have yet to discover the obesity gene and, once found, it may take decades to crack the code. But we already know that obesity and a tendency to be overweight can be inherited or rooted in the behavior we learn from our families. If both parents are overweight, you will have to work a little harder to change your genetic predisposition. Remember from Chapter 1 that if you know you have a family history of easy fat gain, diabetes, or heart disease, you will want to ensure that you don't eat the same way as Mom and Dad, and you will want to think differently, too. You know that it is not just your genetic makeup, the foods you choose, your hormones, or lack of exercise, but also your psychological and emotional programs, that can keep you trapped in patterns of behavior that increase your propensity to overeat and not exercise. And where do all these patterns begin?

BORN WITH OBESITY RISKS

Both the foods your mom ate while you were still in the womb and the foods you were fed during early childhood have an effect on the likelihood of weight problems. If a woman develops gestational diabetes during pregnancy, her baby is at higher risk of having an increased number of fat cells. This is one reason adopted children have been found to have similar body composition and weight-management concerns as their biological parents. Feeding children an excessive amount of food during the first few years of life can lead to too many fat cells.

The study most often quoted on genetic factors was led by Dr. Albert J. Stunkard, a prolific researcher on the subject of obesity. He looked at 540 Danish adults who had been adopted. A comparison of height and weight overwhelmingly demonstrated that the individuals studied were more likely to have the same body weight characteristics as their biological parents than those of their adopted family.

PARENTAL EATING PATTERNS

Other studies have been conducted on the metabolic rate of children. Researchers found that children of overweight parents had a lower metabolism than did the children of parents who were not overweight. We know diets that are predominantly made up of refined carbohydrates (processed cereals, white flour, white sugar, white rice) and low protein lower metabolic rate, so it makes sense that if children eat the same types of foods as their parents, they will also have similar fat-burning rates. But being overweight has more at its core than having an increased number and size of fat cells and overweight parents. Psychologists point to the patterns of behavior that send people down the fat path.

REWARDS, LOVE, AND FAT PATTERNS

Patterns of behavior in children are formed at an early age. Parents, other primary caregivers, and then teachers provide a framework for children about how to behave, and food is often one of the techniques used to reinforce or deter certain behaviors. Frequently children are rewarded with candies, cookies, and junk food for good behavior or to get them to stop a behavior that adults find annoying. A child looking for attention soon learns that along with that attention comes food.

In other words, the child discovers that love and feeling good are associated with eating. Most of us have experienced this, but probably never thought about it. When we are young, a warm chocolate chip cookie is often given to soothe a bad day at school. A beer might make an adult feel good after a hard day at work. Alcoholic beverages are high in sugar. Sugary foods also wreak havoc on your blood sugar balance and serotonin levels. When you eat sugar, your serotonin (the feel-good hormone) increases, and you feel better. Thus there is a vicious cycle of cravings and weight gain. When your mood drops, you suddenly start craving sugar-laden foods or alcohol. Eating these foods causes your serotonin to increase, and you feel good, but when the serotonin level drops, you crave these foods again. Balancing your moods and maintaining normal serotonin levels can reduce food cravings and binge eating.

HOME ALONE SYNDROME

In most families, both parents work and children are often left to fend for themselves before and after school. In an average week most adults spend forty to fifty hours at work, fifty-six hours sleeping, thirty hours doing housework, and twenty-one to thirty hours watching television or searching the Internet. Children between the ages of two and eleven average nineteen hours watching television, and children older than eleven spend twenty-one hours or more on average per week in front of the television. Even families with very low incomes may have on average two televisions.

What's worse, the television sends thousands of negative messages about food. One Saturday morning I watched television with my grandsons, aged seven and five. Within a one-hour period they learned about dozens of different types of fattening, toxic, fast foods and saw endless negative messages. Legislation has stopped cigarette manufacturers from targeting our children, yet fast food restaurants are allowed, without any restrictions, to encourage our kids to eat foods that will cause heart disease, diabetes, and cancer. And these advertisers are slick. It must be hard for parents of young children to say no to determined kids who want a McDonald's Happy Meal™ with the hot toy of the week.

Kids left home alone for long periods or those who have to find their own entertainment choose video games and television and therefore do not get enough exercise. Furthering the obesity problem at a young age is the habit of watching television while eating, a comforting thing to do while waiting for Mom or Dad to come home from work. This is a negative behavior—albeit one that most adults and children are unaware of that comfort can come from the cookie jar or microwave popcorn. Eating the wrong foods, combined with little or no exercise, causes people to pack on weight. I was a fat child and, after school, while my Mom was at work, I could eat through a kitchen full of food.

TIPS FOR FAMILIES WITH CHILDREN

- Remember, *you* purchase the groceries and *you* drive the car. Your children can't eat junk food if you refuse to buy it.
- Purchase washed and cut veggies so they are ready to use when you come home from work or when you are putting lunches together. They will also be ready for kids to eat when you aren't home.
- Stock your cupboards with protein shakes and high-protein power bars that contain healthy ingredients. Don't buy snack cakes and cookies.
- Buy real fruit juice, not soda pop or sugar-laden, artificially flavored and colored water.
- On Sunday, bake lots of chicken (skinless) or boil eggs so they're ready to eat for the next few days. Then it will be easy for you to make lunches with good, clean protein, not bologna and processed meats.
- Limit television and video games to a certain number of hours per day and certain days per week. I know parents who unplug the cablevision before they leave for work. Others put video games under lock and key.
- Sit down with the entire family to eat supper and talk to your kids. If you can't do this every night, then pick a couple nights a week that are mandatory family nights. Too many families are so busy that they fail to teach their children about proper eating habits.
- Play with your children—dance in your living room, go for walks, throw a ball, ride a bike, or just have fun. Spending time with your children in fun activities will stop the negative pattern of television and food consumption that most families have adopted.
- Say loving words to your children every day. Tell them, "Have I told you how much I love you today?" or, "You are so beautiful and smart." And start early—most children learn patterns by five years of age. Good self-esteem is essential to a child's psychological eating habits.

EMOTIONAL HEALING FOR WEIGHT MANAGEMENT

The psychological aspect of being overweight is not my area of expertise, so a dear friend of mine who has been effective at helping me recognize some of my negative patterns has graciously provided his insights into how to undo what we have learned since childhood. The following section is co-authored with Paul Cassidy, Ph.D. He has been blessed by his mentor and personal teacher, Eckhart Tolle, author of the life-changing, best-selling book, *The Power of Now*. Eckhart's guidance and his book on spiritual enlightenment transformed Paul's life. Eckhart taught Paul that incessant, fear-based, negative thinking is the primary cause for most pain and unhappiness.

Paul is an alcoholic, albeit one who has not had a drop of alcohol for more than a decade. Paul met Eckhart Tolle at the right time in his life—when he had hit rock bottom. His marriage had ended, his business was failing, he was very overweight, he had given up on life, and he was contemplating suicide. Eckhart helped him undo the patterns that had led him to this path. Paul was the son of an alcoholic, and he had learned multitudes of negative patterns early in boyhood. With Eckhart's help, Paul learned to listen to the signals his overweight and unhealthy body was sending.

Paul has taught me to smell the roses and see that my own personal issues are all self-made and originate from old programs I learned way back in childhood. Those who have been reading my books and listening to my lectures are probably saying, "What? She has it all together." But I am a workaholic and constantly strive to do better and better, even to the detriment of my health and relationships. You can learn from Paul's lessons too.

Paul's teachings are so basic—we all want to be seen, heard, and loved—so let's start today by loving ourselves, listening to our bodies, and seeing the positives. Focus on yourself. You can fix only yourself. No one else can make you feel good about yourself if you don't. To help you on your path to a healthier body, find a mentor or friend who can help motivate you to get in shape.

Be Present at This Moment

The average human being experiences approximately 60,000 thoughts in any given day. Ninety percent of them are negative thoughts. In other words, we spend most of our waking day in at least a state of unease, if not downright stress. Our focus on the negative lends itself to looking for quick fixes outside ourselves. These fixes can take many forms, among them drugs, alcohol, and food. We are looking for relief from all our negative feelings and thoughts, most of which are associated with relationships, finances, and work.

WHAT IS STRESS?

Although we may not be aware of them, there are many stressors that affect us daily: noise, crowded cities, polluted environments, a lack of exposure to the sun and fresh air, driving, crime, pathogens, a lack of joy in life, abuse, school, work, too much exercising, chronic allergies, lack of sleep, trauma, anger, intense heat or cold, loneliness, and negative thinking.

The first step in identifying your stress triggers is to be very honest. As mentioned earlier, food is often used as a coping mechanism to handle the stresses of everyday life. If you do not face up to what is causing stress, you will continually hide in your coping mechanisms. The first stage is the hardest, so be gentle with yourself; there is no failure on this course.

IDENTIFYING YOUR STRESS TRIGGERS

If, when you think you have a problem, you eat or drink unhealthy foods or do destructive things like watch television to provide relief, then instead follow the steps below to deal with stress and you will be well on your way to a beautiful, healthy body.

THE STRESS RESPONSE

Stressful events prompt the adrenal glands to secrete several hormones. Cortisol, the main adrenal hormone, is responsible for keeping your blood sugar at normal levels to meet all the energy demands of your body. Cortisol decreases insulin sensitivity and glucose uptake and maintains proper levels of blood sugar. When your adrenal glands are fatigued or exhausted, cortisol levels drop below normal, and they are unable to balance your blood sugar. Chronic stress (something most of us experience) causes your blood sugar levels to rise; then you develop insulin resistance, and too much insulin in your blood, so you gain weight and are at risk for syndrome X and diabetes (discussed in Chapter 9).

Adrenal stress hormone (cortisol) also promotes urinary excretion of magnesium. Magnesium, an important mineral that calms nerves and helps you deal with stress, is needed for more than 300 enzymatic reactions in your body, and when it is low, you crave sugars and have terrible mood swings.

You learned in Chapter 1 that cortisol also activates fat cells to store fat and makes the fat cells in your abdominal wall very resistant to fat loss.

The excess weight you carry around your waist may be caused by your stress levels.

Symptoms of Adrenal Fatigue

- You are tired even after eight hours of sleep
- You crave salty foods
- You have no energy
- You feel like you are struggling to do everyday tasks
- You have a low libido
- You can't handle stress
- You need more time to recover from illness, trauma, or grief
- You get light-headed when you stand up quickly
- You feel low or experience mild depression
- You have lost interest in your life
- You get raging PMS (women only)
- Your thinking is fuzzy
- You have memory problems
- You feel like you need to go to bed in the afternoon
- You start to feel awake after dinner
- You have no energy to exercise, and even walking up a few stairs is exhausting

Adrenal Help

The following tips can help rejuvenate tired adrenals.

- Go to bed before 10:30 p.m. and stay in bed as long as you can the next morning. (To aid restful sleep, take 1 to 3 mg of melatonin every night.)
- Do light exercise every day, such as yoga, Tai Chi, stretching, Pilates, and walking.
- Avoid all caffeinated beverages—drink herbal teas like chamomile.
- Use sea salt on your food, and eat kelp and green and black olives.
- Choose foods low on the glycemic index (see Chapter 2).
- Do not eat fruit on its own in the morning without adequate protein as it raises blood sugar and insulin, disrupts serotonin and increases cortisol.

- Include essential fatty acids from flaxseeds, fish, evening primrose oil, or borage oil, and coconut butter.
- Take digestive enzymes with your meals, and chew your food thirty times.
- When exercising, do not push through your exhaustion. If you are tired, stop!
- Take ashwagandha, rhodiola, suma, Siberian ginseng, schizandra berries and a good multivitamin with minerals to help nourish and support the adrenals.

Constant stress promotes adrenal exhaustion and a corresponding drop in thyroid function. When your thyroid is stressed and your thyroid hormones are low, you gain weight and your fat cells become resistance to fat loss. Low thyroid function is discussed in Chapter 2.

Serotonin and Sugar Cravings

We eat, on average, 150 lbs (68 kg) of sugar per person per year. Sugar is not only sweet, it has a powerful chemical effect in the body, commonly called the "sugar high." When we eat sugary foods, our blood sugar levels rise, but sugar is quickly metabolized. Soon after eating it, our blood sugar quickly falls, causing low moods and a feeling of fatigue. Earlier we saw when our happy hormone, serotonin, is low we crave sugar-laden foods. Serotonin is very important: it signals the brain that we are full and satisfied. When serotonin levels drop, we crave more sugar or carbohydrates, starting the cycle all over again.

STRESS TEST TO DETERMINE WEIGHT MANAGEMENT

Check off the situations that apply to you and circle the corresponding number. The following statements determine your happiness level, how you handle stress, and if you have negative thinking.

☐ I am worried about paying my bills this month	1
☐ I look at myself in the mirror and think negative thoughts	3
☐ I am lonely	3
☐ I dislike my job	3
☐ I like my job, but have too much work to do	1
☐ I like my job, but my boss is too demanding	2

☐ I am always trying to please everyone	3
☐ I am exhausted, but keep going	3
☐ Sometimes my stomach feels like it has butterflies in it	1
☐ I shop to make myself feel better	1
☐ I feel guilty or angry	2
☐ I have feelings of inadequacy (not feeling good enough)	3
☐ I am afraid of failure	2
☐ I have feelings of anxiety or low moods	2
☐ I feel trapped; sometimes I think I can't cope	3
☐ I crave sugar	1
☐ I am a single mother	2
☐ I am a university student	1
☐ I am in an unhappy marriage	3
☐ I live with an alcoholic or a drug abuser	2
☐ I work shift work	1
☐ I work too much and don't have enough playtime	1
☐ I get angry with myself	2
☐ I don't eat regularly	
(I wait more than four or five hours between meals)	3
☐ I am sick more than three times a year	1
☐ I lack sexual desire	1
☐ I smoke, or drink alcohol or too much caffeine	2
☐ My family and friends are not supportive of the things I do	2
☐ I am tired all the time	3
☐ I have friends that take, but never give	2

Total _____

How Did You Score?

- If you scored below 15 you are handling stress, but you need to find more balance in your life.
- If you scored from 15 to 30, you know you have to make some changes fast. You are at risk of adrenal exhaustion.
- If you scored more than 30, you are over the top and need to adopt strategies to reduce your risk of stress-related disease.

The stressors mentioned above provide constant, low-grade stress that keeps you in a state of unease, which can lead to unnecessary eating.

STRESS-BUSTING TIPS

- Breathing is a powerful de-stressing tool. Several times per day, breathe in through your nose and fill your lungs with air until your abdomen rises. Then slowly exhale from your mouth until your lungs are empty. Repeat this five times.
- Get eight hours of sleep every night and try to sleep until 7:30 in the morning.
- Learning to say no when you have too much to humanly accomplish in one day is important to healthy adrenals.
- Have the family share the household workload. Doing chores together can be fun.
- Eat plenty of vegetables every day.
- Smile. This chapter will teach you how to purge negative emotions.
- Get help in dealing with grief. The loss of a loved one, a divorce, or the loss of a job all produce grief. Immune suppression is the result when grief is not dealt with.
- *Carpe diem*—seize the day—and live it to the fullest. Don't worry so much about tomorrow.
- Believe in yourself. Negative self-talk and continually doubting your abilities will hamper your body's ability to heal.
- Notice the beauty around you. Smell the flowers, watch the sunset, and listen to the wind.
- Love your family and friends and be forgiving.
- Be good to yourself. Most of us are our own worst enemies. We focus on our weaknesses and minimize our strengths. Wake up each day and tell yourself you are a good and useful person.
- Do the things you have always wanted to do. Learn to water ski, sing in a choir, write a book, tell stories to your grandchildren, walk, garden— whatever makes you happy.
- Seek your spiritual side. This effort does not have to be religious, although those with strong religious beliefs generally live at peace and feel protected. Most of us believe in something greater than ourselves, a spiritual power that offers solace and helps us find the quiet place within.

(*Source*: Reprinted with permission from Lorna Vanderhaeghe, *Healthy Immunity: Scientifically Proven Natural Remedies for Conditions from A–Z*. Toronto: John Wiley & Sons, 2002.)

Create Positive Images

Stand in front of the mirror in the morning and tell yourself how wonderful you are, what a great smile you have, how shiny your eyes are, how strong you look. Do it every day. Surround yourself with motivating images. Then pick up your weights that have been hidden in the bedroom closet and use them. Go for a walk at lunchtime today. Smile at everyone. It is impossible to be negative or unhappy with a smile on your face—just try it! Smiling also enhances your serotonin levels, thus shifting your hormones to a positive state.

Make More Time for Fun

Ask yourself what you are missing—time with friends, going for a walk, a swim at the pool, a sauna, reading a novel, playing games with the kids, kissing your spouse? Make a pact with yourself that once a week you will do something you miss. Then ask what you hate doing—sitting in front of the television, washing laundry, cleaning, driving the kids to a dozen activities, dealing with your boss? Then make a decision to change one thing a week. If you hate your boss, spend every spare moment looking for a new job. Hire a maid, even for one hour a week. Teach the kids to do laundry (they can learn as young as age five to sort clothes). Get call display so you can avoid people who make you feel bad. Understand your life choices—don't do things that make you miserable. Fill your life with positives. Ask yourself how much your life will change if you are healthy and fit.

Negative Self-Talk

North American society is entrenched in negative thinking at a very young age. We hear the word "no" thousands of times by the age of three. Paul has found that the most commonly held belief among those working with him to reframe their lives is the idea that they are not good enough or that they are failures, along with the associated feelings of guilt, shame, and fear. For example, parents separate after years of heated arguments, which often involve the children. The children learn that they are the reason their parents are no longer together, and they feel guilty for causing the breakup. Or parents might compare one of their children to the other. Innocent comments are often filed away in a child's mind and affect self-esteem. Statements such as, "Your sister is so much better at mathematics than you are—you must just not have a head for numbers." These messages often come from those we trust and love the most—our parents, teachers, and friends. We then use these messages to define who we think we are. The result is that we are programmed to deliver what we believe ourselves to be. We know we should change what we eat and exercise more if we want to lose weight and achieve better health. We are intelligent, but we are unable to sustain the changes we know are good for us, so we must stop saying we are fat, ugly, too old, too out of shape. We must retrain our thoughts and believe we are fit, beautiful, and sexy. Say, "I am beautiful, sexy, and fit." Repeat six times while looking at yourself in the mirror. Laugh into the mirror—it feels strange, but don't stop.

Changing Your Program to Reduce Your Weight

Now you know you have a choice. You can choose to continue that old negative thought process or you can start fresh. Paul's technique works. It is simply about positive affirmations and visualization. There is extensive literature on the success of this approach in every facet of people's lives, including weight loss. One of the people who popularized the application of positive affirmations was Dr. Maxwell Maltz, author of *Psycho-Cybernetics*. Dr. Maltz was a famous plastic surgeon. He discovered that many of his patients who had had successful surgery still had feelings of negative self-worth, and that they needed to undergo reconstruction of their psyche to achieve wholeness.

Affirmations

The first step in changing your negative self-concepts is to become present in the moment. It will take practice to become aware of only this moment. Sit in a comfortable chair or lie on the bed. Close the door. Be aware of your breathing, right down to the tips of your fingers and toes. Breathe in through your nose and out through your mouth. Breathe deep into your abdomen. Be aware of any sensations in your body. Follow this by observing the thoughts in your mind. The process is to just be, not to analyze or judge your feelings or thoughts. You will feel calm. Once you feel calm, you will be ready to introduce new ways of thinking, called patterning. It is important to create positive statements, called affirmations, that come from your heart. One affirmation that works well for me is "I deserve to have it all." Here some other positive affirmations:

"I am enjoying my fit and healthy body."
"I am eating healthy and nutritious food in appropriate amounts."
"I drink lots of healthy liquids, especially water."
"I am exercising every day."
"I am a good person."

Note that affirmations are always in the present tense and are always positive. They are designed to teach you to stop thinking negatively, so if you find yourself thinking "I can't stop eating," change it to "I will eat only good, healthy foods."

Visualization

Visualize your new body in the shape and weight you want, and experience the feelings and emotions you associate with the new you. Practice your affirmations and visualizations at least three times a day, preferably more. The changes often start happening within a very short time, but allow six weeks for the new program to be fully operational. You may start noticing, for example, that when you go to the supermarket, you no longer go to the aisle with the potato chips and cookies. You have reprogrammed yourself to realize that junk food is no longer appropriate for who you are supposed to be. You will notice how conscious you are of your thoughts and emotions. Once you become very good at this exercise, you will notice that even if you decide to eat something unhealthy, you will note that it was your choice, not an unconscious act.

A JOURNAL FOR OPTIMAL HEALTH

You need to use tools to support you on your journey. One of those tools is a journal. A journal serves two purposes. First, it helps you be aware of how you are feeling in the moment. Second, it helps you record patterns that identify what is working and/or not working for you. Resistance to journal writing may be overcome by an affirmation such as "I am successfully keeping track of what I eat and how I feel." Remember that your old program will try to stop you from being successful.

Sample Journal

Have a look at this sample journal. If you follow this model you'll learn so much about how your emotions impact your eating habits.

Breakfast

How did you feel before breakfast?

☐ Anxious ☐ Tired ☐ Grumpy ☐ Harassed/stressed ☐ Bored ☐ Satisfied
☐ Excited/enthusiastic ☐ Energetic ☐ Other _____

What food did you eat? What did you drink? _____

_____

How did you feel after breakfast?

☐ Anxious ☐ Tired ☐ Angry ☐ Harassed/stressed ☐ Bored ☐ Satisfied
☐ Excited/enthusiastic ☐ Energetic ☐ Other _____

Mid-morning

What did you do this morning?

☐ Work ☐ Watch TV ☐ Exercise ☐ Social activity
☐ Work around the house ☐ Hobby

How did you feel?

☐ Anxious ☐ Tired ☐ Angry ☐ Harassed/stressed ☐ Bored ☐ Satisfied
☐ Excited/enthusiastic ☐ Energetic ☐ Other _____

What food did you eat? What did you drink? _____

_____

How do you feel now?

☐ Anxious ☐ Tired ☐ Angry ☐ Harassed/stressed ☐ Bored ☐ Satisfied
☐ Excited/enthusiastic ☐ Energetic ☐ Other _____

Midday/Lunch

How did you feel before lunch?

☐ Anxious ☐ Tired ☐ Angry ☐ Harassed/stressed ☐ Bored ☐ Satisfied
☐ Excited/enthusiastic ☐ Energetic ☐ Other _____

What food did you eat? What did you drink? _____

_____

How do you feel now?
- ▣ Anxious ▣ Tired ▣ Angry ▣ Harassed/stressed ▣ Bored ▣ Satisfied
- ▣ Excited/enthusiastic ▣ Energetic ▣ Other _____

Mid-afternoon
What have you done this afternoon?
- ▣ Work ▣ Watch TV ▣ Exercise ▣ Social activity
- ▣ Work around the house ▣ Hobby

How did you feel?
- ▣ Anxious ▣ Tired ▣ Angry ▣ Harassed/stressed ▣ Bored ▣ Satisfied
- ▣ Excited/enthusiastic ▣ Energetic ▣ Other _____

What food did you eat? What did you drink? _____

_____

How do you feel now?
- ▣ Anxious ▣ Tired ▣ Angry ▣ Harassed/stressed ▣ Bored ▣ Satisfied
- ▣ Excited/enthusiastic ▣ Energetic ▣ Other _____

Dinner
How did you feel before dinner?
- ▣ Anxious ▣ Tired ▣ Angry ▣ Harassed/stressed ▣ Bored ▣ Satisfied
- ▣ Excited/enthusiastic ▣ Energetic ▣ Other _____

What food did you eat? What did you drink? _____

_____

How do you feel now?
- ▣ Anxious ▣ Tired ▣ Angry ▣ Harassed/stressed ▣ Bored ▣ Satisfied
- ▣ Excited/enthusiastic ▣ Energetic ▣ Other _____

Evening
What did you do this evening?
- ▣ Work ▣ Watch TV ▣ Exercise ▣ Social activity
- ▣ Work around the house ▣ Hobby

How did you feel?

☐ Anxious ☐ Tired ☐ Angry ☐ Harassed/stressed ☐ Bored ☐ Satisfied
☐ Excited/enthusiastic ☐ Energetic ☐ Other _____
What food did you eat? What did you drink? _____
_____

How do you feel now?

☐ Anxious ☐ Tired ☐ Angry ☐ Harassed/stressed ☐ Bored ☐ Satisfied
☐ Excited/enthusiastic ☐ Energetic ☐ Other _____

Looking for the Patterns

When you examine your journal you will likely start to see patterns of the most challenging behaviors that need to be changed. Perhaps you will note situations at work that regularly trigger stress, and when you are stressed you go to the vending machine and get a chocolate bar. Perhaps when you get home from work you feel guilty that you are a bit late because you were held up in traffic and the kids have had to wait for their supper, or you did not eat all day so your serotonin levels are low, so you start snacking on a bag of cookies while you make the evening meal. When you read your journal, you can see the areas you need to focus on. Sometimes evening is the most difficult time of day to maintain healthy eating habits. If this is the case for you, go to the gym after supper, or take the kids for a walk to the park. If you find the television is your trigger to eat ice cream, potato chips, or other unhealthy foods, then remember to practice your positive affirmations, such as, "I am strong and smart and don't need to eat while I watch television."

TRIGGERS AND AFFIRMATIONS

Now that you know what needs to be changed and when, you can focus on the how. The first step in breaking the old program is to focus on the moment and achieve a sense of calm. Observe your breathing, body, and thoughts. Now recite an affirmation that is part of your new program. An affirmation for your work situation may be, "I am at ease and I am in control." Experience the feeling of being relaxed and at peace. An affirmation for your home life may be, "I am a wonderful, loving parent." Now you will experience feelings of peace and love. Remember to write down several affirmations that work for you.

PRACTICE, PRACTICE, AND PRACTICE

If you want to change what you have been doing in the past, you must practice, practice, and practice. Start your day by reminding yourself and affirming that you are a wonderful, loving human being—that is one of the most important statements you can make. Say it as you wake up, say it in the shower, say it when you go to work or play. If you doubt the efficacy of this approach (your old program does not want you to succeed), then fake it until you believe it by repeating the affirmations over and over! There is plenty of evidence that this does work, so be willing to give yourself a chance.

THERE ARE NO FAILURES

So what happens when you forget to do your affirmations or forget to choose peace when you are stressed? Or you fall off your new eating program? Just start again. It takes time for your new program to kick in and, as with anything else in life, you have to do your apprenticeship. Keep changing your affirmations until you find ones that work for you. Enjoy creating new ones. You will discover other little programs that you have been trapped in. You will then know how to create a new affirmation that will help you overcome them.

TRACKING HOW YOU FEEL AND WHAT YOU EAT

If you have a weakness for sugar, this will become very apparent as you read your journal entries. The journal has been set out so that it is easy for you to record not only what you eat, but how you feel when you were eating and afterward. Once you recognize your behavior, you will see the negative patterns that are keeping you trapped. You will be able to create new affirmations that will enable you to overcome your negative programs. Be very honest with yourself.

YOU ARE NOT ALONE

You are far more likely to succeed in changing eating and exercise habits if you can surround yourself with support. Everyone knows this, but if you are like most people, you may find it difficult to ask for help. Very often people feel they should be able to make changes on their own and are ashamed to ask for help. An easy way to turn this around is to ask yourself how you feel when someone asks you for help. Usually you feel good, respected, honored, and powerful. In other words, when you ask someone for help, you give that person the gift of self-esteem. When you ask your friends, relatives, and colleagues for help, you are giving them the gift.

BE TRUE TO YOURSELF

It is time for you to recognize that you are a gift to all around you. As you turn your life around, you will become an example for others who want to follow in your path. To achieve this, all you have to do is remember the truth of who you are. Before you learned all those negative programs, who were you? You were an innocent child, full of love, joy, fun, and curiosity, exploring the world. It is time to remember that, yes, you now consciously choose to practice your love, joy, and wonder every day of your life.

Celebrate life and imagine each day full of love, joy, peace, and serenity. Remember the excitement of seeing and learning things for the very first time.

Your Hormones and Weight Gain

In Chapter 1, I briefly touched on the hormones that contribute to weight gain. Insulin, cortisol, thyroid, serotonin, and the sex hormones testosterone and estrogen all play a role in either keeping you thin or promoting weight gain. This chapter will examine the reasons these hormones become disrupted and how they affect the way your fat cells work. Hormones are proteins secreted from many glands of the body. They act like messengers and affect thousands of bodily functions. Scientists studying obesity have learned that fat cells secrete their own set of hormones, further compounding the problem of obesity.

FAT CELL FUNCTION

Fat cells (also called adipose tissue) are located in different places in men and women. Men tend to carry body fat in their chest and abdomen. Women carry it in their breasts, hips, buttocks, thighs, and waist. Estrogen and testosterone play a role in the position of fat on the body. And there are two types of fat: white fat and brown fat. White fat insulates you from the cold, cushions your structure, and is a source of energy. Brown fat is very important for producing heat (thermogenesis). Brown fat cells are composed of mitochondria, the energy producers of the body, which generate heat.

There are two types of obesity. In hypertrophic obesity, fat cells are too large. In hyperplastic obesity, there are too many fat cells. The size of your fat cells can change during your life, but the number of fat cells is determined by the time you reach your late teens. The types of foods your mother consumed while she was pregnant affects the number of fat cells you have. If your mother had gestational diabetes, your fat cells are affected. And the amount of food fed to you throughout your childhood also has an effect. During your mother's third trimester of fetal development, and again when you go through puberty, your fat cells form at increased rates. This is why healthy, appropriate childhood nutrition is key to adult weight management.

MORE THAN STORAGE

Scientists around the world have found that fat cells, swollen to capacity, spew out vast amounts of hormones and chemical messengers that hasten death from heart disease, strokes, diabetes, and cancer. Moderately obese people cut their life span by up to five years, and the severely obese see a reduction of at least ten years. Fat cells are now viewed as one of the most important endocrine systems in the body. Approximately twenty-five signaling compounds—including resistin, leptin, adiponectin, inflammatory proteins, tumor necrosis factor-alpha, interleukin-6, growth hormone, and estrogen—send out messages that can promote or attenuate dozens of deadly health conditions.

Doctors used to think that the high blood pressure associated with weight gain occurred because the blood had to be pushed through more mass. Now we know that fat cells can manufacture a potent constrictor of blood vessels, called angiotensinogen; it's a major contributor to high blood pressure in overweight people, whose fat cells are killing them. Combine this blood-constricting hormone with the inflammatory factors produced by the fat cell, and artery walls develop a buildup of tissue that blocks blood flow, increasing the risk of stroke and heart attack.

FAT CELLS AND CANCER

Growth hormone and estrogen produced by fat cells also fuel cancer cells. Obese women are more likely to develop estrogen-dominant cancers, particularly breast cancer, and they are more likely to die from the disease, because their fat cells pump out copious amounts of estrogen. Overweight women who have not gone through menopause yet have an increased risk of developing polycystic ovarian syndrome, ovarian cysts, fibrocystic breasts, migraine headaches, uterine fibroids, endometriosis, and acne, as a result of their bulging fat cells.

Xenoestrogens (estrogen mimickers found in the environment, in plastics, cosmetics, hair dyes, pesticides, PCBs, parabens, glycols, and hundreds of chemicals) are stored in fat cells. Even an extra 10 lbs. (4.5 kg) of fat increases these deadly estrogens, which disrupt hormone balance in the body, congest the liver, and further increase rates of cancer.

Think of the fat cell as an active manufacturing facility of hormones with lots of fat-storage capacity that can maintain its size. As you just learned, size is one problem.

THE YO-YO EFFECT OF WEIGHT GAIN AND LOSS

Since as early as the 1940s, experiments in humans have shown that each person has a programmed set point weight. This is the weight at which your body regulates your appetite by telling your brain, through various hormones, whether you need to eat. When your fat cells shrink during calorie restriction, one of the twenty-five messengers in the fat cells sends powerful instructions to the brain telling it to eat. Once the fat cells are fed and enlarged, this urgent message is most often turned off. Sometimes, though, fat cells become even larger after yo-yo dieting, and your set point becomes higher. People who have dieted for decades know this effect. With each consecutive diet, they get fatter.

Dr. Michael Murray, leading authority on nutrition and author of *How to Prevent and Treat Diabetes with Natural Medicine*, says: "The set point seems to be tied to how sensitive our fat cells are to insulin. Obesity leads to insulin resistance and vice versa. When there is a lack of insulin or if the cells of the body have become insensitive to insulin, it results in diabetes. When cells become insensitive to insulin, not only is the transport of blood sugar into the cells impaired, but there is also impaired burning of fat stores for energy. When fat cells are full of fat, insulin triggers fat cells to make more fat cells. New fat cells send a signal to the brain to eat to fill up the fat cell and the vicious cycle continues. The set point theory explains why diets don't improve insulin sensitivity and most often fail to provide long-term results."

FAT CELLS CONFUSE INSULIN

One of the most prevalent dangers is that oversize fat cells leak fat into the bloodstream, thereby inhibiting insulin's action (see Blood Sugar and Insulin, below). Fat leakage is not just a problem for inhibiting insulin; the leaking fat can end up in the heart muscle, causing congestive heart failure, and in the liver, promoting fatty liver (see Chapter 1). After hepatitis B and acetaminophen poisoning (acetaminophen is a common over-the-counter painkiller), misplaced fat in the liver is the next biggest reason for liver transplant in North America today.

BLOOD SUGAR AND INSULIN

Understanding how insulin functions can lead you to your ideal weight and reduce the risk of developing diabetes and syndrome X, a disorder marked by insulin resistance.

Glucose, also called blood sugar, is the fuel for all cells. Jack Challem, author of *Syndrome X*, calls glucose our "biological gasoline." It's used by all cells as a source of power. Glucose is not the only fuel for the body; amino acids, glycogen (a form of glucose stored in the liver), fats, and ketones (which are made from the breakdown of fats) are also used as sources of energy. Insulin, a hormone manufactured by the pancreas, shuttles glucose from the blood into our cells, where it is burned for energy.

The body requires a constant supply of glucose. Severe drops in blood glucose cause hypoglycemia (low blood sugar); the symptoms are shaking, dizziness, fainting, mood swings, and, in extreme cases, coma. Conversely, too much blood glucose that is not normalized by insulin causes diabetes. Your body protects you most of the time from low blood sugar by telling you to eat, and the liver secretes glycogen to increase glucose levels. With high blood glucose, your pancreas secretes insulin, sending glucose into the cells.

Your glucose level when you wake up in the morning (called fasting glucose) can range from 65–120 milligrams per deciliter (mg/dl). The ideal glucose range is 80–100 mg/dl. Glucose levels naturally rise after you eat, then fall back to normal. The post-meal normal peak is 65–139 mg/dl. People with diabetes often have high levels of fasting glucose or post-meal glucose. If you have a properly functioning glucose system, you'll experience a slight increase in post-meal glucose. Abnormally high glucose levels signal the body to secrete insulin to move the glucose from the bloodstream into the cells. If you have glucose levels that stay high and do not revert to normal levels, you will develop insulin resistance.

Insulin is a hormone involved in metabolism; it also stimulates cells to take up glucose. That glucose provides energy to the cells. Insulin's chief function is to aid the body in storing fat. This was important back in the days when food was in short supply, but today, with an overabundance of food and a lack of exercise, this function is making fat cells fatter.

The standard diet of too much carbohydrate and not enough protein can disrupt the body's ability to regulate blood sugar adequately. When too much insulin is pumped out to reduce abnormally high blood glucose, you inevitably gain weight; you become fat, and your cells become very resistant to insulin and fat loss. Everyone who is overweight has insulin resistance, and insulin resistance puts a person at higher risk of heart disease, cancers, and diabetes. Those who have upper body fat and are shaped like an apple, and those who have a beer belly with excess weight around the middle, are at serious risk of disease. And by now you realize that to lose weight you have to maintain healthy blood sugar and corresponding insulin function. There is a simple way to accomplish this: a unique viscous fiber supplement, found in tablets and meal replacements.

NORMALIZING BLOOD SUGAR AND INSULIN JUST GOT EASIER

Vladmir Vuksan, Ph.D., one of the most respected and recognized experts on the role of diet in diabetes, heart disease, and obesity, developed PGX™ (PolyGlycopleX) after intense research at the University of Toronto. Dr. Vuksan and his colleagues (including Dr. David Jenkins, the inventor of the glycemic index) have conducted extensive research with various combinations of soluble fibers at the Risk Factor Modification Centre at St. Michael's Hospital, University of Toronto.

Dr. Vuksan and his colleagues discovered that by combining various soluble fibers in specific ratios, the viscosity of the fibers was amplified. The improved viscosity is directly related to the fiber's effectiveness in maintaining proper blood sugar balance and insulin regulation. Michael Lyons, M.D., and Michael Murray, N.D., worked cooperatively with University of Toronto researchers to modify their formulation for better stability through the digestive tract and its characteristics as a food ingredient.

PGX's appetite-suppressing and blood sugar-stabilizing properties continue for hours after ingestion. PGX also fills you up, shutting off those messages to keep eating more and eliminating aggressive cravings. When you take it with a meal, PGX lowers the glycemic index of that meal. It allows you to reduce the number of calories you consume in a day, and it ensures that you maintain the ketogenic action of a very low-carbohydrate diet without having to rigidly avoid carbohydrates (see Chapter 2).

Use PGX as a snack to help burn fat. PGX can be added to protein shake mixes, then poured it into dessert cups with a dollop of real whipped cream on top. It makes a yummy, filling dessert that everyone loves. Remember that permanent weight loss requires stabilization of blood glucose and improved insulin sensitivity. Most of the glucose in your body comes from the carbohydrates you eat, so you must eat only the good carbohydrates, not the processed sugars, crackers, cookies, biscuits, bagels, and breads. It is not complicated—eat foods that are as close to their natural state as possible, with lots of variety and in moderation.

PGX lowers after-meal blood sugar levels by approximately 20–40 percent and also lowers insulin secretion by about 40 percent, producing a whole body insulin sensitivity index improvement of 50 percent. No other drug or natural product or diet can do this. PGX also lowers blood cholesterol and triglycerides, both very real problems for diabetics and those with Syndrome X.

SYNDROME X

Syndrome X was first recognized by university endocrinologist Dr. Gerald Reaven. It is characterized by a collection of metabolic abnormalities, including impaired glucose tolerance, high cholesterol, high triglycerides, high blood pressure, low DHEA, high cortisol, depression, and abdominal fat. Elevated insulin and insulin resistance are the underlying factors. Syndrome X is a prediabetic state, where blood glucose is high but not high enough to be diagnosed as diabetes. Research has found that PGX significantly improves all aspects of Syndrome X by increasing insulin sensitivity. PGX reduced total cholesterol by 12.4 percent, "bad" LDL cholesterol by 22.3 percent, the ratio of LDL to HDL cholesterol by 15 percent, and serum fructosamine by 5 percent. In another study, after-meal glucose was reduced by 27 percent, and after-meal insulin levels by 41 percent; insulin resistance improved by about 48 percent.

Causes of Syndrome X

- Aging
- Excessive alcohol consumption
- High-carbohydrate diet
- High sugar intake
- Insulin resistance
- Vitamin and mineral deficiencies
- Processed foods
- Lack of exercise
- Smoking

Healthy foods that slow a blood sugar rise include:

- Lemons, apple cider vinegar, wine vinegars, and balsamic vinegars (but not regular white vinegar). Use liberally: these foods slow the release of glucose and reduce the GI of foods you combine them with
- Raw or slightly steamed vegetables (preferably green)
- Whole grains in their original state
- Free-range meat, free-range eggs, seafood, soy, protein powders, and free-range poultry

Bad foods that make blood sugar skyrocket include:

- Sugar
- White flour, white spaghetti, white rice
- Soft drinks
- Processed goods
- Yogurt sweetened with sugar and fruit
- Fruit, Fruit juices, jams, and jellies
- Jell-O™ and Kool-Aid™
- Alcohol

Eliminate as many of the bad foods as you can.

INSULIN AND STRESS

Another deadly aspect of high insulin is that it increases the secretion of cortisol, the stress hormone. A rise in cortisol causes a drop in the hormone dehydroepiandrosterone (DHEA), which helps increase muscle mass. More muscle increases fat burning and reduces insulin. As you can see, high insulin promotes a cascade of very negative effects.

ADRENAL HEALTH

I discussed adrenal function and its effects on appetite in Chapter 3. Now I will look at adrenal health with regard to excessive stress and resulting cortisol.

Adrenal Glands

The adrenal glands are among the most important organs in the body. These small glands secretes sex hormones and stress-response hormones that guide the entire body's reaction to stress. They are the organs responsible for the front-line work of adapting to stress. Accumulated effects of internal and external stressors profoundly affect your adrenal glands and, in turn, your hormonal health.

You have two adrenal glands, one on top of each kidney. In response to triggers from the brain, the adrenals secrete hormones that permit your body to respond to stress by increasing your blood sugar levels; your rate of breathing; your cardiac output; blood flow to the muscles, lungs, and brain; and cellular metabolism—the famous "fight-or-flight" response. The adrenals are also responsible for producing cortisol hormones, aldosterone, estrogen, testosterone, and many other hormones. These hormones help regulate metabolic, excretory, reproductive, mineral balancing, and immune defense functions.

The secretion of these stress-response hormones is one of the most important functions of the adrenals. These hormones help us adapt over the longer term to the stresses of life; they stimulate the conversion of protein to energy so energy levels remain high even after glucose is used up in the fight-or-flight reaction. Other hormones help maintain elevated blood pressure and help deal with emotional shocks, infection, high workload, weather changes, environmental chemicals, physical or emotional trauma, and so on.

Symptoms of Adrenal Fatigue

When your adrenal glands are under stress and on the verge of exhaustion they provide you with some very clear symptoms. Check any of the following statements that apply to you.

- ☐ You crave salty foods
- ☐ You have insomnia in which you fall asleep, but wake up several hours later and can't go back to sleep
- ☐ You feel exhausted when you wake up in the morning
- ☐ Your fatigue is not improved with sleep
- ☐ You lack energy
- ☐ You feel like you are pushing yourself through the day
- ☐ You have no libido
- ☐ Little stressors make you feel anxious and angry
- ☐ You suffer from recurring infections
- ☐ You have chronic respiratory problems such as asthma and allergies
- ☐ You take longer than you should to recover from sickness
- ☐ You have low blood pressure
- ☐ You feel faint when you stand up quickly from a sitting position
- ☐ You have low moods
- ☐ You lack interest in things that used to make you feel happy
- ☐ You need coffee or other stimulants to give you a boost of energy
- ☐ You have extreme hot flashes, night sweats, or PMS
- ☐ Your memory seems to be failing
- ☐ You feel like you have cotton in your head
- ☐ You are exhausted by walking up the stairs or doing simple tasks
- ☐ You feel like you are dragging yourself through the day, but wake up after dinner
- ☐ Your face and neck look suntanned, but you haven't been in the sun

If you have more than six of these symptoms, do some of the simple tests at the end of the next section.

Cortisol, the Hallmark of Stress

The hormone cortisol is secreted by the adrenal glands in response to physical, psychological, or environmental stress, and is gaining attention as the hallmark of stress. However, cortisol is more than a simple marker of stress levels; it is necessary for the action of almost every function of your body. Excess or deficiency of this crucial hormone can cause a variety of physical symptoms, which, if not treated, can lead to chronic disease or death. Cortisol regulates hormones, glucose metabolism, and the immune system; it also regulates your body's use of proteins, carbohydrates, and fats.

Your ability to adapt to stress depends upon optimal functioning of your adrenal glands and regulation of cortisol secretion.

If you experience chronic stress, your cortisol levels will remain elevated. Research now correlates chronically elevated cortisol levels with blood sugar problems, fat accumulation, the ability of fat cells to become resistant to fat loss, compromised immune function, infertility, exhaustion, chronic fatigue, bone loss, high triglyceride levels, and heart disease. Memory loss has also been associated with high cortisol levels. As you can see, continual stress can indeed have a negative effect on many areas of your health. The extreme end of excessive secretion of cortisol results in Cushing's syndrome.

Long-term elevations of cortisol can cause your adrenal glands to wear out, so they can no longer produce normal levels of cortisol. After this comes adrenal exhaustion, which contributes to conditions such as chronic fatigue syndrome or, in extreme cases, Addison's disease (in which the adrenals do not produce enough cortisol).

The adrenals secrete both male and female sex hormones—androgens and estrogens—and are the prime producers of estrogen and progesterone during the transitional years when the ovaries take a well-deserved rest. The adrenals are also the sole source of estrogen for men. In today's world, most women (and people in general) have some degree of adrenal compromise. Women generally work full-time, raise children, and juggle other demands of daily life. Poor adrenal health directly affects a woman's ability to smoothly make the transition into menopause. Cortisol production has a natural rhythm. Your body produces more cortisol in the morning than in the evening, giving you the energy you need to begin your day. The cortisol levels should drop by 90 percent in the evening as you leave the stresses of the day behind and start to unwind and relax. A recent study found that women who work outside the home and have family responsibilities tend to have elevated evening cortisol levels. Men, on the other hand, have lower cortisol levels in the evenings. The difference may reflect the additional responsibilities women have after they get home from their day jobs (cooking dinner, laundry, and child rearing). The study may explain why more women have difficulty sleeping and losing weight, particularly during the perimenopausal and menopausal years when the ovaries shut down and the adrenals become a major source of estrogen. Elevated cortisol levels at night prevent sleep or cause very light sleep with frequent waking.

Those with adrenal exhaustion tend to overeat in an attempt to bolster their energy levels, which results in weight gain. They often consume plenty of caffeinated beverages and sugar-laden foods in an attempt to get some quick energy. Couple this with the fact that high cortisol levels make fat cells resistant to fat loss and promote deposition of abdominal fat, and those with adrenal fatigue may feel like they are losing an impossible battle when it comes to weight loss. However, there is a way to repair adrenal exhaustion.

Do you need adrenal support? Take these adrenal function tests. Most people are surprised to find that many of their symptoms are related to poor adrenal function.

Adrenal Function Tests

If you answered yes to six or more of the questions in the adrenal symptom chart on page 107, you may want to evaluate your adrenal gland function with the following tests, which are available at your naturopathic or holistic medical doctor's office.

ACTH Suppression Test (also called the Cortisol Suppression Test): This is a lab test commonly used to measure cortisol blood levels. However, results rarely show extreme enough alterations in cortisol levels to indicate a health problem.

Most adrenal conditions are due to suboptimal function of the adrenal glands, and it is difficult to diagnose mild to moderate adrenal compromise by using only a cortisol suppression test; the results will probably fall within the normal range.

Adrenal Stress Index (ASI): An excellent method for assessing adrenal maladapation to stress, the ASI is an accurate and convenient method for assessing adrenal function by testing cortisol levels in the saliva. Saliva cortisol results have been used in stress research for more than ten years.

The body's levels of cortisol vary throughout a twenty-four-hour period. With a home kit you can collect samples of saliva during the day, making it possible to measure the daily rhythm of cortisol production.

Glucose Tolerance Test: There is often a relationship between low blood sugar and low adrenal function. A five- to six-hour glucose-tolerance test can rule out blood sugar irregularities. Any physician can order this test.

Reclining/Standing Blood Pressure: This is an easy assessment of adrenal function. Your blood pressure is measured while you are reclining, then taken twice more when you are brought to a standing position. In a normal response, the blood pressure will be approximately 10 mg/hg higher in the standing position than in the lying position. If you have a low adrenal function, your blood pressure will drop 5 mg/hg or more when you move from the lying to the standing position. With a few exceptions, this test is a reliable indication of the adrenal state.

You can support and treat your adrenal glands with vitamin and mineral supplements and with botanical medicines; also try by balancing workloads, rest, family time, physical and spiritual exercise, and personal playtime. If you believe your adrenals are exhausted, it is important that you employ these solutions to be successful in losing weight.

Adrenal Support Necessary for Weight Loss

Adrenal support is key in your battle to reach and maintain a healthy weight. Let's take a look at a few things that can help boost your adrenal support.

Adaptogens

Herbs that help you adapt to stress by supporting the adrenal glands are aptly called adaptogens. They improve your ability to cope with stress—physical, environmental, mental, and emotional. Adaptogens have many important properties, but the most important is their normalizing effect, regardless of the condition. They help your body maintain homeostasis, the constant internal state necessary for health and life itself. For example, if your blood pressure is high, an adaptogen will help lower it; if it is low, the same adaptogen will help normalize it.

Some of the common health-enhancing and adrenal-supporting functions of adaptogens include:

- improving blood sugar metabolism
- supporting the endocrine (hormonal) system
- protecting and supporting the immune system
- providing liver protection and support
- increasing stamina and endurance
- strengthening the cardiovascular and respiratory systems
- strengthening the brain and central nervous system
- protecting cells from antioxidant damage

Anti-stress Herbs

There are many herbs on the market that can help with stress. Here are a few.

• **Siberian ginseng** (*Eleutherococcus senticosus*): This herb is known as the "King of Adaptogens." It is respected for its ability to support adrenal function and enhance immune function. Studies have demonstrated that it is virtually nontoxic. In Russia, Siberian ginseng is well known for its ability to increase stamina and endurance in athletes. Siberian ginseng can be used to counter fatigue, give immune support, improve decreased mental abilities, and support the body during periods of high physical exertion.

Recommended dosage: Standardized to contain 1 percent eleutherosides, 100 mg one or two times daily.

• **Rhodiola** (*Rhodiola rosea*): This herb is one of the newer adaptogens in North America, but it has been intensively studied for more than thirty-five years in Russia. Russian researchers have observed that rhodiola increases resistance to a variety of chemical, biological, and physical stressors; it also offers antifatigue, antidepressant, immune-enhancing, anticancer, and cardio-protective effects. It improves the nervous system and mental function by increasing blood supply and protein synthesis. Rhodiola is beneficial in the treatment of insomnia, poor work performance, fatigue, hypertension, memory problems, and depression.

Recommended dosage: Standardized to 3.5–4 percent rosavins, 4.5 percent salidrosides, 100 mg one or two times daily.

• **Ashwagandha** (*Withania somnifera*): Ashwagandha is my favorite herb. It is referred to as Indian ginseng and has been used in India's traditional medical system for more than 2,500 years. While numerous studies have explored this herb's ability to improve stress tolerance, combat fatigue, improve memory problems, enhance immune modulation, and benefit inflammatory conditions such as arthritis, recent research has examined its positive effect on people suffering from hormone imbalances and low thyroid function. It is exceptionally important if you have exhausted adrenals and low thyroid function. Ashwagandha is an excellent remedy for nervous system complaints such as anxiety and insomnia.

Recommended dosage: Standardized to 1.5 percent withanolides, 80 mg one or two times daily.

• **Suma** (*Pfaffia paniculata*): Suma is both the common name and the trade name for this plant. In Brazil, it is also called para todo, a Portuguese phrase meaning "for everything." Traditionally it is used as an energy and rejuvenating tonic as well as a general cure-all for many types of disorders. Suma is an excellent herb for the cardiovascular system, central nervous system, reproductive system, digestive system, and immune system. In Europe, suma is commonly used to treat fatigue, menopausal symptoms, impotence and other sexual difficulties, respiratory problems, blood sugar imbalances and diabetes, cancer, and other diseases related to chronic immune deficiencies. It is a source of beta-ecdysterone, which is often used to help athletes increase muscle mass and endurance.

Recommended dosage: 100 mg one or two times daily.

• **Schizandra** (*Schisandra chinensis*): In traditional Chinese medicine, schizandra is commonly used as a general tonic herb to purify the blood and restore liver function. It improves cell turnover, which declines with aging. It is also used as an adaptogenic herb to counter the effects of stress and fatigue. Scientific studies show it has normalizing effects in cases of insomnia, gastrointestinal problems, and immune system disorders. Schizandra improves mental function and enhances physical and intellectual endurance.

Recommended dosage: 80 mg one or two times daily.

Adrenals and Salt

People with adrenal fatigue often have low blood pressure. One of the first symptoms of low adrenal function is salt cravings. The adrenal glands regulate mineral and water balance in the body. Without adequate sodium to make this system function properly, blood pressure drops. Salt will increase blood pressure to normal in those with weak adrenals and restore other cellular functions that require sodium. Many people restrict their salt intake, with two consequences: (1) they are not getting the iodine (in iodized salt) that helps thyroid function, and (2) they are not providing the adrenals with necessary sodium for adrenal balance. Low- to no-sodium diets, which eliminate water weight gain, are not healthy for people with weak adrenal glands. I am not recommending that you consume tons of salt—just be aware that salt is necessary for the adrenals. If you have high blood pressure, avoid salt. Processed, packaged foods are usually full of sodium, but these are not the foods you should be consuming. Most vegetables, especially celery, contain a small amount of sodium. Use sea salt, rich in many minerals. Olives are another good food for the adrenals, as they are naturally salty.

The adrenals are intricately linked to the thyroid gland, and disruption in one gland automatically puts pressure on the other. The effects of cortisol, secreted by the adrenals, on the thyroid gland is shown in the list below.

Elevated Cortisol (stress hormone)
Leads to: ⬇
Weight gain ⬇
Abdominal fat cell enlargement ⬇
Increased cravings for sugar and carbohydrates ⬇
Increases in cholesterol and triglycerides ⬇
Afternoon fatigue ⬇
Desire to eat at night ⬇
Decreased serotonin, the feel-good hormone that stops food cravings ⬇
Memory problems and accelerated brain aging (shrinking hippocampus) ⬇
Increased tumour necrosis factor alpha, Interleukin-6,
    and Interleukin-1, promoting inflammation ⬇
Unbalanced immune function ⬇

Increased aromatase and estrogen in the fat cells ⬇

Sleep problems and reduced melatonin levels ⬇

Low sex drive ⬇

High blood pressure

Low Thyroid Function (metabolism hormone)

Elevated cortisol uses up tyrosine, which is used by the thyroid gland to make thyroid hormone and ensure that it is converted from T4 to T3 (the more active thyroid hormone).

Leads to: ⬇

Decreased ability to burn fat ⬇

Morning aches and pains ⬇

Weight gain ⬇

Stubborn weight loss resistance ⬇

Exhausted adrenals ⬇

No sex drive ⬇

Heavy periods ⬇

Memory problems ⬇

Hormone problems (hot flashes, night sweats, mood swings) ⬇

Infertility and recurring miscarriage ⬇

Estrogen belly fat

The result is the inability to lose weight and keep it off.

THE THYROID–ADRENAL RELATIONSHIP

If there is inadequate thyroid hormone, the adrenal glands are affected, and if there are inadequate levels of some of the adrenal hormones, the thyroid does not function properly. The adrenal–thyroid feedback interaction is orchestrated by the nervous system.

Earlier I mentioned that your adrenals are your main stress-adaptation gland. When your adrenal glands are overworked, your body converts progesterone (a precursor hormone) into adrenal hormones. This depletes the progesterone you need for other functions, such as bone health and balance of estrogen. Both the thyroid hormones and progesterone have a normalizing, anti-stress effect on the pituitary. Thus they help the adrenals—which, like the thyroid, are stimulated by the pituitary—with stress adaptation. When progesterone levels fall because progesterone has been converted into stress-fighting hormones, the thyroid suddenly has to take on the task of removing stress from the body.

Furthermore, the thyroid governs your metabolic rate, the rate at which you burn fat for fuel. If the adrenals are depleted, the thyroid will whip them into order, hormonally speaking, to maintain the proper rate. However, the endocrine system does not continue this strategy forever. Instead, over time, the thyroid decreases hormone production to conserve adrenal energy (and its own). When this first happens, you may have symptoms of both adrenal and thyroid imbalance. If the symptoms are not addressed, over time they will come to be predominantly related to one gland or the other—most often the thyroid.

THE THYROID GLAND

The thyroid, located at the front of the throat, sets the rate of body metabolism, regulating every cell in the body. Therefore, any change in thyroid functioning will have far-reaching effects. The following hormones and substances directly affect the thyroid or are released by it:

- Thyrotropin-releasing hormone (TRH) is secreted by the hypothalamus, a brain center that coordinates the actions of the nervous and endocrine systems. TRH triggers the pituitary to secrete the thyroid-stimulating hormone (TSH).
- Thyroid-stimulating hormone (TSH) is secreted by the pituitary and stimulates the production of thyroid hormones and the growth of thyroid cells. Too much TSH causes enlargement of the thyroid.
- Calcitonin is a thyroid hormone involved in the balance of blood calcium levels. It lowers the amount of calcium and phosphate in the blood as necessary by inhibiting bone breakdown and accelerating the absorption of calcium. A healthy thyroid gland is essential for strong bones. If you have osteoporosis, get your thyroid checked.
- Thyroxin (T4) is the most abundant thyroid hormone and is manufactured in the thyroid gland. It is made from tyrosine and iodine.
- Triiodothyronine (T3) is the most active thyroid hormone, with four to ten times the activity of T4. Twenty percent of T3 is produced and secreted by the thyroid gland, and the other eighty percent is converted from T4

115

in the liver and other organs. Many factors contribute to the conversion of T4 to the more active T3, including a healthy liver, your stress levels, and the types of foods you consume.

At any given time, most T3 and T4 molecules in your body are bound tightly to proteins in your blood. Only small amounts of each circulate as "free" hormones—the active hormones that can turn on or off the cellular functions necessary for controlling your metabolic rate (the rate at which you burn fat). For example, unbound T4 accounts for approximately 0.05 percent of the total amount of T4. Free hormone levels are seldom measured by medical doctors, yet these levels provide the most accurate way to determine thyroid function. In a free T3 hormone test, the normal range is 2.3–4.2. A result of less than 2.3 indicates low thyroid function. In a free T4 thyroid hormone test, the normal range is 0.7–2.0. A reading of less than 0.7 suggests low thyroid function. Request free thyroid hormone tests along with the TSH.

Low thyroid function causes body functions, particularly the regulation of body fat, to slow down. The symptoms of low thyroid function can be subtle (slow weight gain, constipation, gradual thinning of the hair) and may appear slowly over time (see symptoms, below).

Severe hypothyroidism, confirmed by a thyroid-stimulating hormone test, requires the use of thyroid medication. Most medical doctors prefer the synthetic thyroid hormone, T4, but some physicians and patients prefer desiccated natural thyroid obtained from the glands of animals (mainly pigs). Desiccated thyroid also contains the more active T3 thyroid. It may be difficult to find the correct dose of desiccated thyroid medicine unless your doctor is willing to monitor your TSH, T3, and T4 closely with the blood tests mentioned earlier. (This is a problem in Canada, where medical doctors are not familiar with natural hormones and where the medical system will pay for only certain diagnostic tests and only so many per year.) Desiccated thyroid is available through compounding pharmacies in Canada. Compounding pharmacies belong to a group of pharmacies that specialize in the latest techniques in pharmacokinetics. The Professional Compounding Consultants Association can be reached at 1-800-331-2498.

Thyroid and Hormone Problems

It is common for the thyroid to be out of balance in women who experience hormone-related problems such as premenstrual syndrome (PMS), infertility, ovarian cysts, fibroids, endometriosis, fibrocystic breasts, menstrual pain, heavy bleeding, or severe menopausal symptoms (particularly hot flashes and night sweats). Back in the days before fertility drugs, when a woman could not get pregnant or had recurring miscarriages, doctors prescribed thyroid hormone to facilitate a pregnancy. Women who suffer postpartum depression may also benefit from thyroid hormone, as childbearing can often exhaust the adrenals and cause low thyroid function.

Hypothyroid or low thyroid hormone is a common condition in North America, particularly in Canada and the northern United States, where sunlight is low and soil mineral depletion is common. Low thyroid function affects approximately 20–25 percent of the female population and about 10 percent of males. Thirty percent of people older than thirty-five may have mild hypothyroidism: their TSH is within normal range, but they have many of the symptoms of low thyroid function. The thyroid secretes two hormones, T3 and T4, which are crucial for controlling your metabolism. Because thyroid hormones affect every cell in the body, a deficiency will result in many symptoms.

Symptoms of Low Thyroid Function (Hypothyroidism)

- Cold hands and feet, cold intolerance, low body temperature
- Constipation
- Chronic fatigue, weakness, lethargy
- Edema (swelling of eyelids or face)
- Depression and irritability; sudden change in personality; nervousness
- Hair loss; dry, coarse skin, hair, or both; cracking in the heels and skin
- Hormonal imbalances (uterine fibroids, ovarian or breast cysts, infertility, miscarriage, painful periods, endometriosis, heavy periods, PMS, menopausal symptoms, frequent menstrual cycles)
- Impaired memory; poor concentration
- Slower metabolism, which may show up as weight gain, either general or on the hips
- Shortness of breath; inability to breathe deeply

- Enlarged thyroid gland (goiter)
- Headaches and dizziness that are worse in the morning, but better in the afternoon
- Heart palpitations
- Insomnia; racing thoughts
- A metallic taste in the mouth; this symptom indicates a need for iodine
- Poor vision
- Terrible menopausal hot flashes and night sweats that do not abate with treatment
- Slow Achilles reflex (see home thyroid tests)
- Low basal temperature (see home thyroid tests)
- High TSH: Low T3, T4, or T7, or a presence of thyroid antibodies
- Carpal tunnel syndrome
- Elevated cholesterol levels
- Low progesterone-to-estrogen ratio
- Recurring miscarriages and infertility
- Slow pulse

Mild Low Thyroid Function

Many people's thyroid blood test (TSH test) falls within the accepted parameters for normal (0.3–6.0 IU/ml). Some thyroid experts believe that the range for normal is too broad and that, as a result, too many people are not being treated for this common condition. Most people with levels greater than 2.0 IU/ml but less than 5.5 IU/ml have symptoms of low thyroid function. Enlightened doctors say such people have "subclinical" or "functional" low thyroid function. If you are trying to lose weight, and you have followed a healthy eating plan and exercised, and if you still cannot lose a pound, you may have subclinical low thyroid function.

You may experience symptoms for up to ten years before thyroid hormone levels drop low enough to result in a mainstream diagnosis of low thyroid function. In the meantime, you will go through much unnecessary suffering.

Diagnosed Hypothyroidism

Conventional medical doctors diagnose hypothyroidism (underactive thyroid) only when TSH levels are higher than 6.0. High TSH levels indicate low thyroid because the pituitary is trying to stimulate the thyroid into action by pumping out more TSH.) This allows for a very broad definition of what is normal.

Many people who have all the signs of low thyroid function may never receive appropriate treatment because the traditional lab tests are insensitive to early changes in function. Abnormal TSH, T3, or T4 levels are rarely found in the multitude of patients with low thyroid function. To confirm a diagnosis of functional thyroid imbalance, caring doctors will also use the following diagnostic tools.

Laboratory Tests for TSH, T3, and T4: The normal range for the TSH test is so broad that most patients who have symptoms but are still functioning are not diagnosed using this test, yet it takes very little change in TSH to cause dramatic changes in thyroid function. It is a mystery that the current definition of the normal range for TSH is so wide, given the extreme sensitivity of the thyroid to even minute variations in TSH levels.

In Canada most doctors test only the TSH level. This is because of financial constraints of the national health plan. If a TSH level is within the normal limits, further thyroid tests are not performed. Yet it is quite common for patients to have normal levels of TSH and T4 but low T3 levels. T4 is the most abundant thyroid hormone (fifty times more T4 is present in the body than T3), but T3 is far more active. Many people are unable to convert T4 into T3 at the rate needed, and will continue to experience symptoms of low thyroid function even when they take medication that normalizes TSH levels. This is because the medication does not increase the T3 level. For additional information on T3, please refer to Dr. E.D. Wilson's book *Wilson's Syndrome: The Miracle of Feeling Well*.

Basal Temperature Home Test: Monitoring the basal temperature is the most sensitive and accurate way to evaluate thyroid function. It's is also the simplest and least expensive test. The thyroid sets the thermostat for the body and regulates the rate of metabolism in nearly all the cells. Therefore, the most reliable window on thyroid function is the basic body temperature, or basal temperature. It is measured at the same time every day—as soon as you wake up in the morning, before arising.

The research on basal temperature as the most accurate measurement for thyroid function was done by Dr. Broda Barnes, who has more than forty years of clinical experience with thyroid patients. Look for two of the doctor's books: *Heart Attack Rareness in Thyroid-Treated Patients* and *Hypothyroidism: The Unsuspected Illness.*

Basal Body Temperature Thyroid Test

Your basal body temperature—the temperature of your body at rest—is the most sensitive test of thyroid function. Note: Menstruating women must perform the test only on the second, third, and fourth days of menstruation, because female hormones affect body temperature, and readings from these days will be the most accurate. Men and postmenopausal women can perform the test at any time.

Take the test as soon as you wake up: it is important to take your temperature after you have had adequate rest. Before you go to sleep, if you are not using a digital thermometer, shake down a mercury thermometer to below the 95ºF (35ºC) mark and place it in an empty cup with the mercury end down by your bed so it will be ready in the morning. Immediately upon waking, before you get out of bed, place the thermometer in your armpit (hold for 5 minutes if you are using a mercury thermometer). Hold your elbow close to your side to keep the thermometer in place. Read and record the temperature and date. Repeat the test for three consecutive mornings (preferably at the same time). A reading between 97.6ºF and 98.6ºF (36.4ºC and 37ºC) is normal. Readings below 97.6ºF (36.4ºC) may indicate hypothyroidism.

Iodine Home Test: Purchase some topical iodine at the local pharmacy. Before you go to bed, apply it to an area of the body (the inner arm works well). Make sure it dries before you put your pajamas on, and leave it on overnight. Doing this test at night is good because in the morning, after eight to ten hours of sleep, you will see the dramatic difference in the color of the iodine swab from the time of application. If the iodine is absorbed by morning (if the color of your skin is normal), you may have a thyroid function problem.

Nutrients to Support Thyroid Health

Several nutrients can improve and normalize thyroid function for people with mild low thyroid function. Also, if you are taking thyroid medication but are still plagued by the symptoms of low thyroid function, you may not be converting the T4 hormone to the more potent T3 hormone, and you will also benefit from these nutrients:

- Potassium iodide
- Tyrosine
- Ashwagandha
- Guggal
- Pantothenic acid
- Vitamin D
- Minerals

Potassium Iodide

To produce thyroid hormones, the thyroid gland needs iodine. A chronic lack of iodine in the diet produces an underactive thyroid gland, which in severe cases causes an enlarged thyroid gland (called a goiter). In North America, salt manufacturers add iodine to table salt, so the incidence of goiters is rare. But many people are avoiding salt in their diet, and they may experience an enlarged and underactive thyroid. Too little iodine in the diet results in impaired thyroid function, while too much interferes with the thyroid gland's ability to produce hormones. Iodine deficiency also promotes infertility and recurring miscarriage; it also causes reduced mental capacity in the offspring of women who are iodine-deficient while pregnant.

Recommended dosage: 50–100 mcg one or two times daily. The dosage range for iodine from all food and supplement sources is 300–400 mcg per day. Read the labels of your food supplements to find out how much you are already taking.

Tyrosine

Tyrosine, an amino acid found in red meat, dairy products, eggs, almonds, beans, avocados, and bananas, is another essential nutrient for manufacturing thyroid hormones. Tyrosine can be made by another amino acid, called phenylalanine, using iron. But many women, especially those in their forties who have uterine fibroids and/or very heavy periods, are often iron deficient. They such cannot make tyrosine and may end up with low thyroid function. People who experience much stress use more tyrosine to deal with the stressors, which can lead to low thyroid hormone output. Low thyroid hormone leads to low blood pressure, cold hands and feet, and restless leg syndrome (in which the legs never feel relaxed and must be moved constantly).

Recommended dosage: 250–500 mg one or two times daily.

Ashwagandha

Ashwagandha (*Withania somnifera*) extract is used in traditional Indian medicine to support the thyroid gland. Studies show that it enhances thyroid function and produces a significant increase in T4 thyroid hormone. It also works with guggal to improve the conversion of T4 to the more active T3.

Recommended dosage: 75–150 mg one or two times daily. Use a standardized form that contains 1.5 percent withanolides.

Guggal

Guggal (*Commiphora mukul*) extract supports complete thyroid health and enhances the conversion of T4 hormone to the more potent T3. Guggal and ashwagandha should always be used together, as these two herbs exert synergistic effects on the thyroid gland. Both herbs appear to boost thyroid function without influencing the release of the pituitary hormone TSH. This means the herbs work directly on the thyroid gland and other body tissues to exert their effects. According to Michael Murray, N.D., 95 percent of all cases of hypothyroidism are due to a problem with the thyroid gland itself and not the pituitary or an impaired conversion of T4 into T3 in tissues outside the thyroid gland.

Recommended dosage: 50–100 mg one or two times daily. Make sure it is standardized to 3 percent guggulsterones.

Other Nutrients

Pantothenic acid supports the adrenal glands, increases energy, helps you handle stressful situations, and reduces cellulite and water retention.

Recommended dosage: 50–100 mg one or two times daily.

Copper and **manganese** are necessary cofactors for the manufacture of thyroid hormone 250–500 mcg of copper and 250–500 mcg of manganese.

Thyroid Medication and Nutritional Supplements

If you are using thyroid medication and your dosage of medication keeps getting increased but you still have symptoms of low thyroid function, the nutrients mentioned above will aid the conversion of T4 thyroid hormone to the more active T3. Thyroid medication is potent. When your dosage is continually increased, your risk of osteoporosis increases. Take these nutrients when you take your thyroid medication. **Do not use these nutrients instead of your thyroid medication. These nutrients are to be used with thyroid medication.**

Sunshine Vitamin and More Minerals

I have mentioned this throughout the book, but I will say it again: Take a good multivitamin with minerals and essential fatty acids as the foundation for your nutrition. Add other nutrients as needed. A multivitamin is especially important for healthy thyroid function. Make sure your multivitamin contains at least 400 IU of vitamin D, which is essential to the manufacture of thyroid hormones. Earlier I said people who live in the northern United States and Canada have a higher incidence of low thyroid function. This is because they do not get enough sunshine throughout the year, and exposure to sunshine is how people manufacture vitamin D. Even in the summer, most people avoid the sun or apply sunscreen to reduce the risk of skin cancer. As a result, they do not make enough vitamin D for adequate thyroid function. Combine that with mineral-depleted soils and water, and low thyroid function becomes a widespread problem. If you live in an area where sunshine, especially in the winter months, is low, then the only way to get adequate vitamin D is to take it in a vitamin supplement.

Thyroid Hormone Treatment

Poor control of thyroid hormone therapy can lead to weight gain. Not enough T4 thyroid hormone combined with poor conversion of T4 to T3 results in an inability to lose weight or causes weight gain in people who are on thyroid hormone. People who have had their thyroid surgically removed because of overactive thyroid or an autoimmune disease also tend to gain excess weight when only T4 is provided without adequate T3 thyroid hormone.

Exercise for Low Thyroid Function

Exercise is particularly important for low thyroid function as it stimulates the thyroid gland and increases metabolism. Exercise daily for ten minutes. See Chapter 7 for simple exercises to jump-start thyroid function.

Diet and Low Thyroid Function

The most important diet changes if you have low thyroid function are to reduce or eliminate the bad saturated fats and trans-fatty acids (see Chapter 2), which inhibit the manufacture of thyroid hormone, and to increase the good essential fatty acids from fish, flaxseeds, olive oil, coconut oil, and nuts and seeds.

Eating more protein is important for adequate thyroid hormone. Protein contains amino acids, including tyrosine, which are essential for the manufacture of thyroid hormone. Eat free-range chicken, eggs, and beef along with nuts, seeds, fish, beans, and legumes.

Increase the amount of vegetables you eat, too. This may seem confusing because some vegetables are antithyroid, also called goitrogens, meaning "to cause a goiter." Vegetables from the cabbage family can inhibit production of thyroid hormones when eaten raw in large amounts. Many nutritionists tell people with low thyroid function to avoid all broccoli, Brussels sprouts, cauliflower, cabbage, and kale. But the truth is you would have to eat 3–5 cups (750–1250 mL) of any of these vegetables raw every day to inhibit production of thyroid hormones. These vegetables, when eaten raw, contain high amounts of thiocyanates; the thiocyanates are reduced when the veggies are cooked or lightly steamed. These vegetables have powerful abilities to protect you against breast cancer and prostate cancer. The warning against them is blown out of proportion.

Foods such as rapeseed (used to make canola oil), cassava (a starchy root, the source of tapioca), maize, sweet potatoes, lima beans, soy, and pearl millet have been listed as foods to avoided if you have hypothyroidism. But only soy has been proven to promote hypothyroidism. Soybeans contain phytates, which bind to the minerals necessary for the production of thyroid hormone. So avoid regular soybeans used in commercial soy milk and in thousands of soy-based foods. But when soybeans are fermented, the phytates are deactivated. Fermented soy is an acceptable food for the thyroid. Fermented soy is found in tempeh, miso, soy sauce, some soy powders, and soy yogurt (see Chapter 5).

The mineral selenium is essential to balanced thyroid hormones. Include in your diet foods rich in selenium, such as Brazil nuts (one of the richest sources), wheat germ, tuna, shellfish, beef kidney and liver, sunflower and sesame seeds, garlic, onions, kelp, and eggs.

The Body Sense Natural Diet is based on a balanced and healthy eating plan, so while you are losing weight, you are supporting proper thyroid hormone function.

LOW THYROID FUNCTION, PERIMENOPAUSE, MENOPAUSE, AND WEIGHT GAIN

Estrogen determines body fat distribution. In women, fat is stored on the hips, bottom, abdomen, and thighs. Fat cells manufacture and store estrogen. Some researchers believe that women get more body fat around menopause to ensure adequate estrogen from fat cells. Others believe low thyroid function and exhausted adrenals promote midsection fat gain. Considering that excess fat reduces life expectancy, I tend to believe the second theory. The body is generally programmed to ensure survival, and too much fat causes heart disease, diabetes, breast cancer, and increased death rates.

I mentioned earlier that as many as a third of people older than thirty-five may have subclinical low thyroid function. Low thyroid function promotes many hormonal problems that could be remedied with thyroid-supporting nutrients or medication (thyroid hormones).

During the perimenopausal years (the ten to fifteen years before menopause) and menopause (one year with no periods), it is common for women to suffer a multitude of hormonal complaints. Hot flashes, night sweats, and sleep disturbances are common. Many people think these symptoms are associated with a decline in estrogen, but the symptoms, especially night sweats and insomnia, are also the hallmark symptoms of low thyroid function. Most menopausal women are given hormone-replacement therapy with estrogen for these symptoms. Perimenopausal women who are still menstruating may be put on the birth control pill. The problem with these treatments is that estrogen further shuts down the thyroid: high estrogen levels interfere with the thyroid hormones, particularly the utilization of T3, the most biologically active thyroid hormone. Too much estrogen—from hormone-replacement therapy or produced naturally—impairs thyroid function.

Many women have gained 10–15 lb (4.5–7 kg) and noticed increased blood pressure after they start taking synthetic estrogen at menopause. This happens because estrogen is an antagonist to thyroid hormone; it slows down the metabolic rate. As the metabolism slows, many women develop difficulties with fat metabolism. This happens because one of the functions of the thyroid hormones is to stimulate fat cells to burn fat. Weight-control problems result.

In addition, serum cholesterol or triglyceride levels may increase. Thyroid activity can also be inhibited by high levels of androgens (male sex hormones) circulating in the blood. Depression and fatigue are the most common thyroid symptoms in menopausal women. Read my book, co-authored with Karen Jensen, N.D., *No More HRT: Menopause Treat the Cause*, for non-hormonal solutions for menopause symptoms. This book covers everything you ever wanted to know about women's hormones and how to correct their imbalance.

Antidepressants and HRT Make Us Fat

Medical doctors frequently mishandle the treatment of menopausal symptoms, prescribing antidepressants, hormone replacement therapy, or both. There has been a moderate decline in the use of hormone replacement therapy since the Women's Health Initiative study in 2002 was halted because of serious safety concerns for the 15,000 women using the combination of synthetic estrogen and progestins (Premarin™ and Provera™, Prempro™). The study found an increased risk of stroke, heart attack, breast cancer, blood clots, memory problems, and more. Now some doctors prescribe antidepressants as a solution to hormonal problems. If someone is truly depressed, medication may be the answer. But for people who need hormone balancing, antidepressants are not the route to follow. Furthermore, antidepressant medication causes weight gain, night sweats, and low libido, many of the symptoms women are being treated for in the first place.

In 1993, Dr. Frank Tallis reported in the *British Journal of Psychiatry* that up to 14 percent of the patients referred to him for depression or some other emotional disorder had subclinical low thyroid function. Once the hypothyroidism was treated, the emotional cloud lifted. I think subclinical low thyroid function is so pervasive that we should be treating it in most women as a first-line defense against hormonal dysfunction.

The adrenal glands of menopausal women work harder. They must help women cope with life's ordinary strains and also with all the emotional and physical stresses that accompany the menopausal transition. The adrenals must begin to provide the sex hormones once produced by the ovaries. Some herbs and nutrients support adrenal function and can be very important to women's well-being during menopause.

Years of chronic stress eventually cause low adrenal function, but before to the organ is compromised, there are usually periods of adrenal overactivity that, if left untreated, result in low adrenal function. Some people, however, stay in the overactive state for a prolonged period. In the mid-1970s, Raymond Peat, Ph.D., pointed out that menopausal symptoms resemble the symptoms of Cushing's syndrome, a disease related to overactivity of the adrenal cortex. For example, hot flashes, night sweats, and insomnia—common menopausal symptoms—are also symptoms of Cushing's syndrome.

CONCLUSION

For many of you, this chapter has provided a new perspective on why you are overweight or obese. You now know you have to control your blood sugar to maintain healthy weight. You can do that by using low carbohydrate, high-protein diets along with PGX to ensure proper insulin action and maintain control over cravings and appetite.

Low thyroid function is a main reason for weight gain, and for the inability to lose that weight once you have put it on. You can support the thyroid by eating healthy food, eliminating bad fats, taking nutrients and herbs, and reducing stress.

The adrenals and the thyroid are directly connected. Treat your adrenals with respect. Get rest, eat good food, reduce caffeine intake, relax, and avoid stress. The stress hormone cortisol makes you fat and alters your fat cells so they resistant weight loss. Stress reduction is paramount.

Women entering menopause should think twice about using estrogen replacement therapy. Too much estrogen inhibits thyroid hormone, thereby promoting weight gain.

The good news is that once you balance these important hormones, the fat will just melt away. Your energy will return, so exercising will be easier. The Body Sense Natural Diet program helps with weight loss and helps eliminate many of your hormonal problems.

Digestive Health

We've covered a lot of ground so far, and now you likely know more about how your body works than you ever have before! In this chapter we'll review how your digestive system functions and how to optimize its performance; we'll learn about the powerful link between digestive health and achieving your weight loss goals. There is no doubt that a healthy digestive system is essential to proper weight loss. If you are not digesting food properly, your abdomen swells, you retain fluid, your food cravings become uncontrollable, and your hunger hormones become confused. In previous chapters you learned that the hormones secreted by the adrenals, thyroid, liver, and fat cells can keep you slim or make you fat. Your liver is the key organ in this battle, as it processes most of your hormones. It is also intimately connected with your digestive system and is the guardian or sentinel organ of the body. Most important for weight loss, the liver interacts with the pancreas to manage your body's glucose and insulin levels.

Now I will have a look at powerful new research showing that the gut (the digestive tract, also called the gastrointestinal tract) secretes its own hormones, many of which conspire to make you fat. Digestive distress caused by leaky gut syndrome, food allergies, *Candida albicans* yeast overgrowth, *H. pylori* (a bacteria that causes ulcers and cancer), or poor eating habits can contribute to weight gain and obesity. You must eat and properly digest the foods recommended in the Body Sense program to reduce the amount of false fat you are packing around. It's called false fat because although it looks like excess fat around the middle, it is actually excess water. If you are suffering from digestive problems, your gut may be sending confusing signals to your brain, causing you to eat uncontrollably and crave carbohydrates. Ultimately, weight loss is inhibited.

SYMPTOMS OF DIGESTIVE DISTRESS

Digestive complaints are so common that many people think they are normal. We have all experienced the odd bout of heartburn, nausea, diarrhea, gas, bloating, burping, and constipation when we have eaten something out of the ordinary or traveled to another country. But when these symptoms become regular, they signal more serious intestinal problems. Check off the following symptoms of digestive distress to evaluate the health of your gut.

- ☐ You develop flatulence, belching (gas), and bloating after most meals.
- ☐ Your lower abdomen is distended, and your stomach sticks out even when you haven't eaten for hours.
- ☐ You get heartburn or indigestion more than once per week.
- ☐ You feel nauseated when you take your vitamins on an empty stomach.
- ☐ You are not hungry when you wake up in the morning after not eating for ten hours.
- ☐ Your skin is sensitive to eczema, hives, acne, or breakouts.
- ☐ You are not having at least one 12-in (30 cm) bowel movement or three 4-in (10 cm) bowel movements per day.
- ☐ You have diarrhea alternating with constipation.
- ☐ You develop abdominal pain after eating.
- ☐ You have bad breath.
- ☐ You feel uncomfortably full after eating a normal-size meal.
- ☐ You have itching around the rectum.
- ☐ You have hemorrhoids.
- ☐ You have weak, peeling, or cracking fingernails.
- ☐ You have broken capillaries around the nose and cheeks.
- ☐ You have age spots on your face and the back of your hands.

▫ You have offensive body odor.
▫ You have varicose veins.
▫ Your tongue is coated with a white substance.

If you have any of the symptoms, you must correct the underlying abnormalities in your digestive tract so you can absorb and digest your food better. Then the hormones of your digestive tract can do their job properly to help keep you slim. Varicose veins and hemorrhoids are a sign of poor elimination. A white-coated tongue is a sign of *Candida albicans*, which can inhibit absorption of nutrients and shut off hormones that tell your brain you have eaten enough. If you are not hungry after sleeping all night, the hormones that turn your hunger signals off and on are disrupted. If you have age spots or broken capillaries in the skin, your liver may not be functioning at peak performance. All these symptoms contribute to weight gain and will cause resistance to weight loss until you correct the situation. This chapter will help you understand what role your digestive system plays in weight management. It will provide you with solutions that quickly correct gut problems. I will examine all the hormones and peptides in the digestive tract and describe how these affect your appetite. I will also describe the environmental triggers that disrupt these hormones, including foods, infections, and stress. I will tell you how to repair the key hormones and peptides that normalize your gut.

HORMONES OF THE GUT

Gut derived hormones and peptides send strong signals to tell the brain when your body requires more food or when it has had enough to eat. Peptides, on the other hand, consist of two or more amino acids that can also function like hormones, help make up proteins, and aid the digestive process. More than two dozen hormones and various peptides have been identified in the gut. The most important regulators of appetite include cholecystokinin (CCK), ghrelin, neuropeptide Y (NPY), and peptide YY (PYY3-36).

• The pancreatic hormone CCK acts on messengers that tell you when you have had enough food to eat. Whey protein powders stimulate and enhance the production of the hormone, which also tells your gallbladder to contract and your bowels to move.

- Ghrelin is secreted by cells in the stomach when you are hungry. The secretions stimulate you to eat. In other words, ghrelin makes your stomach growl. It also suppresses the utilization of fat in fat cells. PGX fiber helps turn off ghrelin and makes you feel satisfied.
- Leptin, another hormone, signals your brain to tell you to stop eating, that you are full.
- Neuropeptide Y is a feeding stimulant that causes storage of your food as fat.
- Peptide YY (PYY3-36), secreted by cells in the intestine after you eat, tells the brain to stop eating and suppresses appetite. Human studies have shown that injections of PYY3-36 caused participants to eat less over a twelve-hour period; the people were noticeably less hungry. The amount of PYY3-36 secreted is determined by the number of calories ingested—the more calories consumed, the more PYY3-36 is released.

How do you get your gut to secrete the right hormones at the right time so you feel full, don't eat too much, and maintain a normal weight? Professor Stephen Bloom, from Imperial College Hospital London, has found that bulky, fibrous foods such as vegetables, which move farther down the gut before they are fully digested, stimulate the secretion of PYY3-36 and tell us we aren't hungry anymore. Fast foods, on the other hand, are dissolved mainly in the stomach and do not enhance the secretion of this peptide. Very soon after eating these foods, you feel hungry again. Avoid fast foods, and eat lots of high-fiber foods to enhance the production of this important peptide.

Whey protein powders signal the body that you are satisfied and no longer require more food. Whey protein also contains tryptophan, which the brain uses to manufacture your feel-good hormone serotonin (see 5-HTP in Chapter 6). The hormone helps reduce sugar cravings. Another component of whey protein powder is lactoferrin, an antioxidant, a powerful antiviral, and an antibacterial agent shown to inhibit the growth of *E. coli*, salmonella, and *Candida albicans* in the gut. Whey protein is a key component of the Body Sense Natural Diet program for these reasons and more.

PGX soluble fiber (see Chapter 4) also fills the digestive system, turning off hormones that make you eat and signaling the brain that you are full.

Probiotics such as *Bifidobacterium* BB536 (sold in capsules), along with foods like lactic acid-fermented sauerkraut, yogurt, miso, and fermented soy powder, help maintain proper levels of friendly bacteria in the gut and prevent an overgrowth of *Candida albicans*. *Candida* can disrupt your gut hormone signals and make you crave foods, especially refined carbohydrates.

LEAKY GUT SYNDROME

Further aggravating the problem of abnormal functioning of your gut hormones is leaky gut syndrome. Years of food allergies, bacterial overgrowth, *Candida* overgrowth, and stress, among other factors, can cause inflammation of your digestive tract. Eventually the delicate tissues are damaged, and openings or gaps occur. Substances can leak through these gaps into the bloodstream, causing leaky gut syndrome (LGS). When waste, bacteria, and partially digested food are allowed to pass into the bloodstream from a damaged or leaky gut, the immune system mounts an assault against these foreign invaders. A leaky gut must be healed quickly, not only to stop the leaking of foreign substances into the bloodstream but also to quell the aggressive immune responses that accompany this condition. Leaky gut promotes the following: food allergies, cramps, diarrhea, bloating, heartburn, weight gain, and autoimmune or other chronic inflammatory disorders.

To heal a leaky gut, avoid the foods you are allergic too, eat healthy foods, take digestive enzymes and probiotic supplements (sold at the health food store), reduce the stress in your life, and chew your food well before swallowing. The gut lining is regenerated approximately every four days, so healing does not take that long if you avoid the saboteurs (white sugar, alcohol, poor food) and the allergens that are causing the problem.

WATER WEIGHT GAIN

Food allergies alone can cause the body to retain as much as four percent of its body weight in water. (This water retention is called edema.) A leaky gut allows toxins into areas of your body where they normally would not be. These toxins then overload your body's organs, especially the liver, which is the key organ in maintaining proper balance of the hormones that manage your weight.

Breaches and inflammation in the intestinal wall also make absorption of nutrients very difficult. The inability to absorb nutrients is called malabsorption, which causes deficiencies, which in turn cause further stress on your body. B vitamins must be absorbed adequately; they produce stomach acid to break down your foods. If your foods are not broken down properly, you will experience gas, bloating, an inability to fight off yeasts, bacteria, and viruses creating further digestive problems. If your gut is not absorbing nutrients, weight gain is inevitable, because you will feel constantly hungry due to nutritional deficiencies.

Malabsorption syndrome occurs when food is not broken down properly or when inflammation in the small intestine is so severe that nutrients cannot be absorbed. Once malabsorption sets in, the most wholesome diet in the world will not prevent nutritional deficiencies; you will need extra supplementation while the gut is healing.

MAGNESIUM

Although every nutrient is important for the optimal functioning of the body, some nutrient deficiencies are very harmful. Magnesium is required for 350 different enzymatic actions, so its deficiency can affect every part of your body. Minerals require carriers to help them across the walls of the intestine into the bloodstream. If you have leaky gut, these carriers are often damaged, and minerals are not absorbed at the optimal rate. Some researchers suspect that up to eighty percent of the population could be deficient in magnesium. Look at the label of your multivitamin and mineral supplement, and make sure you are taking at least 250 mg of magnesium daily.

SOME SIGNS OF DEFICIENCY OF COMMON NUTRIENTS

You have just learned that nutrient deficiencies can make you crave foods. Here is how your body tells you about those deficiencies.

- *Iron*: anemia, sensitivity to cold, digestive disturbances
- *Thiamin, vitamin B1*: a feeling of pins and needles in the feet and/or hands, anorexia, constipation, reduces pain threshold
- *Vitamin B2*: sore tongue, cracks at the sides of the mouth
- *Vitamin B12*: no moons on your fingernails (the white part, in the shape of a moon, at the base of the fingernails, not including your thumbnails); anemia; pins and needles in your feet; heart palpitations (irregular heartbeat)

- *Vitamin D*: bone loss, hypothyroidism, burning mouth and throat, diarrhea
- *Calcium*: bone loss, brittle fingernails, periodontal disease, depression, weight gain
- *Folic acid*: anemia, restless legs (when your legs don't seem to be comfortable unless you move them), digestive problems
- *Selenium*: dry skin, poor immune function, high cholesterol
- *Zinc*: acne, baldness, brittle nails, white spots on nails
- *Protein*: peeling nails, grooves on nails, water retention

HOW GUT PROBLEMS START

Long-term antibiotic therapy can start the process of digestive distress, as can the use of nonsteroidal anti-inflammatory drugs (NSAIDs), which are sold for pain and inflammation of many conditions, including arthritis. Other prescription drugs can injure the gut lining. Food allergies that are ignored can also promote serious gut imbalance. Processed foods, eating on the run, and excessive stress make it more likely that you will develop digestive problems. North Americans buy more laxatives and antacids than any other population in the world, because we have such terrible digestive health. Poor digestion is a vicious cycle as: some of the causes of leaky gut and malabsorption syndrome, such as allergies and *Candida* overgrowth, are also the end result of leaky gut. (See Detriments to Digestion.) If you check off even a few boxes, you need to adopt the strategies in this chapter to correct digestion. Then you will be able to lose weight and keep it off.

Detriments to Digestion

What causes these symptoms to occur? Check any of the following statements that are applicable to you.

- ☐ Improper eating habits, such as rushing to eat and not chewing your food completely before swallowing
- ☐ Insufficient friendly bacteria in the digestive system due to an excess of bad bacteria in the gut from poor food choices (sugar)
- ☐ Insufficient water intake, resulting in hard stool
- ☐ A diet of low-fiber, highly refined foods
- ☐ High sugar consumption
- ☐ Low stomach acid and insufficient digestive enzymes
- ☐ Sedentary lifestyle or lack of exercise

- Emotional upsets and stress
- Bacterial infections (like *H. pylori*)
- Antibiotic use
- Yeast overgrowth caused by *Candida albicans*
- Nonsteroidal anti-inflammatory drug use
- Food allergies
- Frequent air travel across time zones
- Ignoring the urge to go to the toilet
- Vitamin and mineral deficiencies
- Repeated use of antacids, laxatives, or enemas

CONSTIPATION AND WEIGHT GAIN

Constipation is a common problem compounded by both leaky gut syndrome and *Candida albicans* overgrowth. Poor bowel habits (you do not set aside time each day for proper bowel movements) or a diet low in fiber can promote constipation. When your bowel is full of feces, excess toxins inflame the intestinal lining. These toxins interfere with digestion and elimination and promote water weight gain. Constipation puts stress on your liver, which must continue to detoxify the contents left sitting in the bowels for too long. All this causes weight gain. If you are packing around 10 lb. (4.5 kg) of waste material that should have been eliminated, your abdomen will become distended, and you will feel heavy and lethargic—and just think of the toxins in that waste!

Healthy Transit Time

How long food stays in your digestive tract—called transit time—determines how quickly you lose weight. Food should be in your stomach for two to four hours, in the small intestine for three to five hours, and in the colon for ten hours or more. The optimal transit time for food to get from your mouth to evacuation is twenty-four to thirty hours. Most North Americans have a transit time of more than forty-eight to ninety-six hours.

Solutions for Constipation

Adequate fiber consumption is important. Fiber adds bulk to stools and moves waste through the digestive system. The Body Sense Natural Diet is rich in fiber from fresh vegetables. If you are using the meal replacement containing PGX fiber, constipation will not be a problem. The following recommendations will quickly remedy any constipation problems you are having:

- Take at least 250–500 mg of magnesium daily. Magnesium is a natural stool softener.
- Take digestive enzymes with each meal and snack. They help break down your food and ease elimination.
- Use a natural fiber supplement, preferably organic.
- Take 3000 mg pharmaceutical-grade fish oil or, if you are vegetarian, 3000 mg borage, flaxseed, or evening primrose oil.
- Take a probiotic supplement to ensure adequate friendly bacteria in the gut. These bacteria are necessary for movement of waste through the digestive tract. (See Restoring Friendly Bacteria).
- Use herbs, including buckthorn and cascara, to stimulate the contraction and evacuation of waste.
- Make time to go to the bathroom in the morning.
- Elevate your feet while you are on the toilet. The higher the better. You want to get close to the position of squatting.
- Walk thirty minutes every day, or do ten minutes of rebounding daily (a rebounder is a small, low trampoline).
- Use castor oil packs on your abdomen. Take six squares of flannel, wet them with castor oil, place them on your lower abdomen, and put a hot water bottle wrapped in a towel on top; then rest.

For more information on gut problems from pancreatitis to ulcers, see *Gut Solutions* by Brenda Watson, N.D., and Leonard Smith, M.D. This is a fabulous, comprehensive book on digestion.

Digestive Enzymes

Enzymes are catalysts that accelerate certain tasks and make things work faster. Thousands of enzymes and enzymatic reactions keep you alive. Enzymes are involved in blood clotting, immune function, repair to damaged tissues, removing toxins, controlling of excessive inflammation, and more. Enzymes work constantly in the body, like an orchestra playing a symphony with perfect mastery. And enzymes are essential to breaking down your food. You have three basic food materials—proteins, fats, and carbohydrates—and so you need three groups of enzymes.

- Protease enzymes break down proteins.
- Lipase enzymes break down fats and lipids.
- Amylase enzymes break down carbohydrates.

The fresh fruits and vegetables you eat provide enzymes that help you digest your food. Bromelain, the most common enzyme sold in the health food store, is found in naturally ripened pineapples. Asian cultures have eaten enzymatically alive foods for generations. Tamari and soy sauce are some of the oldest enzymatically alive foods. Worcestershire™ sauce is an English example. Choose foods rich in natural enzymes: lactic acid–fermented sauerkraut, yogurt, fresh vegetables, and miso soup.

Find a digestive enzyme supplement that includes a combination of the enzymes mentioned above in capsule form, and take capsules with each meal to aid digestion. Some people may just need a small amount of hydrochloric acid to aid digestion. Betaine hydrochloride is also available in capsules. Start with one capsule until adequate digestion is obtained. You will know when you have achieved this goal when you no longer experience gas, bloating, indigestion, and constipation. If you get a feeling of heat in your stomach when you take betaine hydrochloride, you are taking too much. Cut back.

Look for multivitamins and minerals that contain betaine hydrochloride in their foemula to ensure adequate breakdown of nutrients. Gas and bloating will be reduced and bowel movements will improve quickly when you use digestive enzymes or hydrochloric acid.

CANDIDA ALBICANS OVERGROWTH

Candida albicans is one of many *Candida* fungi, or yeast, that exist in the intestinal tract and skin; in women, it is also found in the vagina. It resides quite peaceably in the intestines and the genital area unless there is an imbalance in the environment that allows *Candida* to grow out of control. When *Candida* proliferates, you can get a yeast infection. Such infections can occur in many areas of your body, including the throat (thrush), nails (fungal infections), bladder (*Candida* cystitis), and vagina (yeast infection).

These infections can affect men as well as women, but women are four times more likely to suffer *Candida* overgrowth. There are approximately 250 species of yeast; the major species that grows in humans is *Candida albicans.*

Candida and Toxic Estrogen Load

Candida organisms can produce hormones, including estrogens and steroids. Also, some types of *Candida* have receptors for hormones on their surface. Receptors are like a lock that needs a key to activate certain signals. *Candida*-derived hormones disrupt gut messages sent to the brain about when and how much to eat and when to stop eating. They also increase our estrogen load, which then inhibits thyroid performance and creates weight gain and health problems. Most people with *Candida* overgrowth have some serious nutritional deficiencies, most likely because the gut is damaged and cannot absorb nutrients. If you suffer from chronic *Candida* overgrowth, you probably cannot lose weight and you may continually crave carbohydrates, a favorite food of *Candida.*

There are more than fifty symptoms that indicate *Candida* overgrowth in the body, including weight gain, sensitivities to chemicals, allergies, asthma, mood swings, fatigue, headaches and migraines, muscle pain, rectal itching, irritability, dizziness, depression, insomnia, and lack of concentration. *Candida* overgrowth has been associated with low stomach acid. Stomach acid is necessary for the breakdown and assimilation of the nutrients in your food; intestinal disorders (including diarrhea and constipation, cramps, and foul-smelling stool, breath, and urine) are very common in those with low stomach acid. The symptoms of *Candida* overgrowth are so similar to other illnesses they can be misdiagnosed. Vaginal yeast infections are apparent by the presence of a white, cheesy discharge with a distinct odor, itching, irritation, and painful urination. Men may also experience genital *Candida* as a urinary tract infection or as an itching or burning sensation at the head of the penis. Dark circles under the eyes, a thick, white coating on the tongue, and fungal infections around the nails are signs of *Candida* overgrowth.

Candida becomes invasive in the body when there are not enough "good" bacteria in the gut. These good bacteria are harmless microorganisms that inhabit the intestinal tract to maintain health. Antibiotics are the best-known culprits that kill the good guys in the gut and allow a hospitable environment for *Candida* overgrowth. Birth control pills, steroids, and chemotherapy can also contribute to the problem. Food allergies, alcohol, dairy products, and diets low in fiber and high in sugar and refined carbohydrates are a smorgasbord for yeast. They can also create the perfect environment for excessive *Candida*.

CANDIDA QUESTIONNAIRE

The following questionnaire will help you discover if you have a *Candida albicans* overgrowth contributing to your inability to lose or gain weight.

General History

Give a score of 3 for each yes answer to the following questions.

___ Have you taken tetracyclines (e.g., Minocin™) for acne for one month or longer during your life?

___ Have you taken, or do you take, antibiotics for infections more than four times per year?

___ Have you taken birth control pills for more than six months?

___ Have you taken Prednisone™ (an immune-suppressing drug) or other cortisone-like drugs (e.g., asthma medication)?

___ Do the smells of perfume, tobacco, or other odors or chemicals make you sick?

___ Do you crave sugars and breads?

___ **Total Score**

Symptoms

Enter 2 if symptom is mild, 4 if moderate or frequent, 6 if severe or constant.

___ Do you experience vaginal discharge or irritation?

___ Do you experience frequent bladder infections or incontinence?

___ Do you experience premenstrual syndrome or fluid retention?

___ Have you had difficulty getting pregnant?

___ Have you had frequent infections (sinus, lung, colds)?

___ Do you have allergies to foods or environmental substances?

___ Do you feel worse on rainy and snowy days, or when you are a round molds or in musty basements?

____ Do you experience anxiety and/or irritability?

____ Do you have nightly insomnia?

____ Do you experience gas and bloating?

____ Do you experience constipation or diarrhea?

____ Do you have bad breath?

____ Do you have difficulty concentrating or do you feel spacey?

____ Do you experience muscle weakness or painful joints?

____ Do you have chronic nasal congestion or postnasal drip?

____ Do you feel pressure behind or irritation of the eyes?

____ Do you have headaches more than once per week?

____ Do you feel unwell without an explanation or diagnosis?

____ Do you have low thyroid function?

____ Do you have no or low libido?

____ Do you have muscle aches or weakness?

____ Do you crave sugar?

____ Do you crave breads?

____ Do you crave alcoholic beverages?

____ Do you crave vinegar?

____ **Total score from all sections**

Scoring:

50 or less indicates mild *Candida*, which is easily treated with a diet change and probiotics.

50–90 indicates moderate *Candida*, which can produce extensive symptoms and inhibit weight loss.

90–120 indicates severe *Candida*, which can lead to some very serious health conditions. You must immediately adopt a strict nutritional program. Eliminate all the bad carbohydrates and employ an arsenal of *Candida*-destroying nutritional supplements.

Candida's Dangers

Yeast's metabolic wastes enter your bloodstream. Your liver has to detoxify these substances in your blood, and becomes stressed. The toxic waste by-products of yeast metabolism also spread to other areas of your body, causing a multitude of symptoms and conditions. *Candida* is accompanied by the proliferation of bacteria that ferment foods, creating gas and toxic compounds, which can indirectly increase your body's total estrogen levels. Too much estrogen contributes to weight gain and a congested liver promotes a cascade of events that make you overweight.

Poor digestion contributes directly to *Candida* overgrowth. Without a healthy digestive process, you will suffer increasingly from nutrient deficiencies and from an increased toxic load (a result of undigested food particles). Your immune system is forced to react to partially digested foods, which it recognizes as foreign substances. When the immune system is busy destroying toxic undigested food particles, its ability to fight disease-causing yeasts and microbes becomes impaired.

Bowel health is central to a healthy hormonal system and weight loss. However, your bowels may be contaminated with toxins that can leach into your bloodstream. Toxins form in the bowel for a number of reasons; among the most detrimental are poor-quality foods. Another cause of bowel toxicity is known as "scanty evacuation." Many people do not understand how they could have a toxic colon when they have "regular" bowel movements. It is shocking that people believe "regular" could range from once a day to once every two weeks. And what is a normal bowel movement? A healthy digestive system produces at least one 12-in (30 cm) bowel movement or three 4-in (10 cm) bowel movements per day. If you work toward this goal, most diseases could be eliminated along with your waste matter. (See solutions for constipation earlier in this chapter.)

TREATMENTS FOR A HEALTHY DIGESTIVE TRACT

The following treatment for *Candida*/intestinal problems is very effective and easier to follow than some of the more restrictive programs. There are four components to the treatment used for cleansing the bowel and decreasing the toxic overload:

1. Make dietary changes to starve *Candida* and harmful bacteria.
2. Cleanse the bowel of harmful micro-organisms and accumulated toxins.
3. Restore beneficial "good" bacteria.
4. Build up your immune system.

Candida Healthy Intestine Diet

The objective of this diet is to reduce the intake of foods that encourage the growth of harmful yeast and bacteria. You will find that these recommendations for healing foods and harmful foods are the same as the Body Sense Natural Diet program.

Foods to Avoid

- Sugars of all types and foods that contain refined or simple sugars
- Dried fruits (raisins, prunes, and dates), which are high in fruit sugar
- Fruit juices, both fresh and frozen (except lemon juice)
- Yeast breads, pastries, and other baked goods (alternatives include yeast-free crackers or rice cakes, sprouted breads, and yeast-free and sugar-free breads)
- Alcoholic beverages
- Processed and smoked meats
- Peanuts. They commonly contain a mold called aflatoxin, which aggravates intestinal problems
- Cow's milk, use only in moderation on cereal or in coffee. Ice cream is a food to avoid. Alternatives include soy, almond, rice, and goat's milk

Foods to Eat Freely

- Fresh, hormone-free meats, poultry, fish, soy foods and fermented soy and/or whey proteins (not sweetened with fructose or artificial sweeteners)
- Eggs
- Raw nuts (except peanuts; see above) and seeds
- Cold-pressed, unrefined flaxseed, coconut and olive oil
- Low-carbohydrate vegetables: green leafy vegetables like chard, kale, celery, lettuce, spinach; broccoli, cabbage, and Brussels sprouts (see glycemic index, Chapter 2)
- Organic butter and yogurt (unless you are allergic to dairy products)

Foods to Eat Cautiously

- Organic fruits—eat no more than one serving per day
- Cereals and other whole-grain products; these should always be yeast-free and sugar-free; choose from the low-carbohydrate list in Chapter 2
- High-carbohydrate vegetables (potatoes, carrots)

Candida Nutritional Products

- Caprylic acid, a fatty acid, is a powerful antifungal. It is produced by the body in small amounts and extracted from coconut and palm oil. Caprylic acid is effective in treating *Candida* overgrowth and intestinal imbalances.
- Oil of oregano in capsules or liquid is a powerful anti-*Candida*, antifungal, antiviral, and antibacterial. The liquid has a very strong taste, so you may want to use capsules.
- Grapefruit seed extracts, taheebo tea, and garlic kill unfriendly microbes.
- Psyllium seed is a bulking agent that helps eliminate toxins by encouraging regular bowel movements and by binding with stored waste products that normally are not eliminated.

Colonic Cocktail Recipe

2 tsp	natural fiber supplement	10 mL
1 cup	water	250 mL
1/2 cup	vegetable juice	125 mL
1 tbsp	caprylic acid	15 mL

Mix natural fiber supplement with water and juice to make it palatable. (Look for organic fiber supplements at the health food store.) Then add caprylic acid.

Drink this mixture once or twice daily, morning or evening, followed by a glass of water. Add a few drops of oil of oregano to the water to increase the destruction of *Candida*. Oil of oregano has a very strong taste, so you can take it in capsule form if you desire.

Drink the cocktail daily for at least six weeks, then drink it twice weekly for another four weeks.

Efficient bowel elimination is essential to normalizing *Candida* balance. Elimination can be encouraged with the herbs buckthorn (*Rhamnus cathartica, Rhamnus frangula*) and cascara sagrada (*Rhamnus purshiana*). These herbs increase the muscular contractions of the bowel, thereby assisting in the removal of toxins. See complete list of constipation remedies on page 137.

Restoring Beneficial Bacteria

The two most important friendly bacteria in our bodies are *Lactobacillus acidophilus* and *Bifidobacteria*. Both are found in good-quality yogurt. In the intestines, they inhibit the growth of unfriendly organisms. These friendly bacteria reduce estrogen reabsorption, the risk of estrogen-dependent diseases, and estrogen imbalance related to weight gain.

Lactobacillus and *Bifidobacteria* are found in fermented foods in cultures around the world. Fermented foods include yogurt, fermented soy powder, miso, tempeh, keifer, lactic acid-fermented sauerkraut, and fermented juices. These foods benefit human health. So do supplements called probiotics, which contain beneficial bacteria. North Americans do not regularly eat fermented foods, with the exception of yogurt. Unfortunately, the friendly bacteria in yogurt usually include little, if any, *Lactobacilli*. Using a high-quality *Lactobacillus acidophilus* and *Bifidobacterium* (BB536) supplement will provide colonization of the friendly bacteria. Look for foods that include fructo-oligosaccharides (FOS), such as asparagus, garlic, onions, and artichokes. Inulin, found in the sap of some roots, is also a good source of FOS. FOS feeds the friendly bacteria, particularly Bifidobacteria, once they are in your gastrointestinal tract, and is not absorbed by the intestines. (See Appendix for recomendations of probiotic supplements.)

Probiotic with Punch

Bifidobacterium longum BB536 has been extensively researched for the past thirty years. It has been proven to prevent and treat *Candida* yeast infections and replenish the good bacteria after you use antibiotics. It supports your immune system and lowers cholesterol levels. And it reduces *E. coli* infection (responsible for urinary tract infections) and prevents diarrhea and constipation. BB536 is shelf stable, so it does not require refrigeration, and it is has the highest counts of friendly, good bacteria in a supplement. Eat foods that are high in friendly bacteria and take a daily supplement to maintain adequate levels of the friendly microbes. Look for nutritional supplements containing BB536.

Now that your gastrointestinal tract is well on its way to optimal functioning, it is time to consider your liver. It is probably feeling better already, since the health of the bowel has an enormous influence on the health of the liver.

THE LIVER: THE GREAT DETOXIFIER

The liver is a remarkable organ and the central chemical laboratory in your body. It is a critical organ in three areas of physical functioning:

- Metabolism
- Blood filtration
- Bile production

Metabolism and the Liver

The liver plays an important role in metabolism. Metabolism uses energy to break down materials in your body and build up substances that form tissues and organs. The most important metabolic function of the liver is the detoxification or inactivation and excretion of toxic chemicals, drugs, and hormones, both those made by the body and those that come from outside sources. The liver renders these substances inactive; eventually they are excreted by the bowels, lungs, kidneys, or skin. The liver is also involved in fat, carbohydrate, and protein metabolism and vitamin and mineral storage.

Blood Filtration

The liver is a major blood reservoir and filters more than 3 pints (1.4 L) of blood per minute. It removes bacteria, toxins, and various other unwanted substances from blood.

Bile Production

Every day the liver manufactures and secretes approximately 2 pints (1 L) of bile. Bile is necessary for the absorption of fat-soluble material (including many vitamins) from the intestines, and the secretion of bile helps your body eliminate many toxic substances.

According to traditional Chinese medicine, the thyroid is also influenced by the liver. The liver energy governs the flow of fluids through the body. When the liver is congested or stagnant, swelling occurs. This swelling may occur in the thyroid area. A noticeable enlargement of the thyroid is a sign of liver congestion. The liver is related to all hormonal imbalances and contributes to being overweight. Liver health is essential to proper functioning of all the hormones that keep you thin or conspire to make you fat.

Stress promotes exhausted or weak adrenal glands (see Chapter 3), which contribute to weight problems. Now you know that stress causes liver dysfunction as well. The three critical organs to effective weight loss are the adrenals, the thyroid, and the liver. Many factors determine whether the liver performs its critical functions well. Too much pressure on the liver from overeating, too much rich or poor-quality food, environmental stresses, overwork, and emotional stress can cause liver overload, and liver overload leads to a decreased ability to clear toxins and hormones and manufacture bile. An overloaded liver allows toxic and waste material to pass into the blood. These toxins accumulate in the body instead of being eliminated.

The Liver and Hormones

Let's consider the pathway the liver uses to clear away estrogens and other hormones, as well as many other compounds. Excess estrogens promote weight gain and low thyroid function, so you need your liver to process your hormones properly.

The liver pathway is the circulation of substances from the liver to the small intestines and bowel and back again. How well this pathway functions determines whether your estrogen and other hormone levels stay balanced. How does this work? Substances, for example hormones, are altered or broken down in the liver and excreted into the bile. The liver secretes the bile into the small intestines. Much of this bile and its load of excreted substances will be eliminated in the feces. If you have an imbalance of friendly and unfriendly bacteria in the gut, or if you suffer constipation, some of the hormones excreted by the liver into the bile may be reabsorbed through the walls of your small and large intestines. These reabsorbed hormones return to the liver via a group of veins. The veins are also responsible for bringing nutrients from food in the digestive tract to the liver for processing. Any disruption of the liver circulation pathway contributes to increased levels of hormones and chemicals in the body.

Too Much Estrogen

The liver is responsible for coupling estrogens and other steroid hormones, certain drugs, and many chemical compounds in the bile for safe elimination from the body. A decreased rate of estrogen excretion through this process may result from liver overload and bowel toxicity. The liver's ability to form combined estrogens may also be decreased if you lack nutrients, for example niacin, vitamin B6, magnesium, methionine, and cysteine. Even mild liver dysfunction may lead to enough decrease in estrogen elimination rates to disrupt hormone balance.

Liver dysfunction is not the only thing that prevents successful estrogen clearance. Bowel health is another key to this process. After the liver forms coupled estrogens, it excretes them in the bile and into the small intestine. These estrogens must stay in their original form throughout the entire length of the intestinal tract to be eliminated in the feces. Think about this process as having the toxins and estrogens wrapped up in a package until they are removed from the body. If elimination time is too long or if *Candida* is present, there will be an increase in gastrointestinal bacteria that break apart the coupled estrogen. Once separated, the estrogen is once again biologically active and is reabsorbed into the bloodstream. Then it must be processed by the liver all over again. Such reprocessing promotes weight gain and the inability to lose weight, along with a long list of female hormonal problems. (For more information on everything you ever wanted to know about women's health and hormones, read my book, coauthored with Karen Jensen, N.D., called *No More HRT: Menopause Treat the Cause*.) However, there are ways to control the estrogen reabsorption. One way is to dramatically cut back on red meat intake. Eating meat raises the level of the enzyme that breaks apart the estrogen couple in the gut. The plant nutrient indole-3-carbinol (I3C) assists in safely eliminating excess estrogen from the body. Eat at least two vegetables daily from the indole-rich family: broccoli, cauliflower, Brussels sprouts, cabbage, kale, and collards. Calcium-D-glucarate, another nutrient that aids the safe removal of estrogen, is found in all fruits and vegetables.

Now that you have a sense of how important the liver is to maintaining proper hormone function and detoxification, you need to look more closely at how to create healthy liver function.

Sluggish or Congested Liver

A person with a congested or sluggish liver may not have liver problems significant enough to cause elevated liver enzymes or other signals detected through standard laboratory tests. Yet the effects of liver congestion, in particular on hormonal health and weight gain, are easy to detect with the following signs and symptoms: estrogen belly (a layer of fat that sits on the abdominal muscles), fatty deposits on the whites of the eyes, yellowing of the whites of the eyes, age spots on the backs of the hands and the face, anger and emotional outbursts, weight gain, gas, bloating, burping, and irritable bowel.

Some of the possible causes of liver congestion include:

- Dietary stresses: saturated fats, refined sugars and grains, low-fiber foods
- Excessive use of alcohol and tobacco
- External toxins from the environment: chemicals and hormones found in food, water, and air
- Internally generated toxins, including those originating from the intestines (discussed earlier)
- Drugs: antibiotics, diuretics, and synthetic hormones, including Premarin, Provera, birth control pills, steroids, and many others
- Obesity
- Type 2 diabetes
- Viral hepatitis, mononucleosis
- Hereditary disorders

Although congestion is a functional condition rather than a pathological one, it can create a variety of physical, emotional, and mental symptoms, ranging from headaches, indigestion, and obesity to bouts of anger and depression.

To detoxify and support a congested liver, start with the simple dietary and lifestyle measures (outlined below) and see how they make you feel. If you feel your liver needs further support, begin using herbs that support liver functions (discussed below).

Lifestyle and Food Support for the Liver

- Start your morning with fresh-squeezed lemon juice in water. This drink helps flush and decongest the liver and stimulates digestion.
- Eat fresh, organic vegetables regularly. Include broccoli, Brussels sprouts, cabbage, dandelion greens, cinnamon, garlic, legumes, and onions.

- Eat green foods and drink green drinks regularly to aid in liver cleansing. Look for these or use a combination of wheat grass juice, dehydrated barley grass juice, chlorella, and spirulina. These can be purchased ready-to-make from your health food store.
- High-quality protein foods are necessary to restore and sustain the liver. Free-range eggs, fish, raw nuts and seeds, and whole grains are beneficial. Eating calves' liver or chicken livers is also beneficial, but make sure the animal was organically raised. Remember what the liver does—it cleanses and detoxifies.
- Antioxidants such as vitamin E, zinc, and selenium are essential for protecting the liver. Take a good multivitamin with minerals daily.
- Liver restoration also requires lots of fresh air, exercise, adequate rest, love, natural foods, and good water.

Liver-Support Remedies

Several herbs have a powerful healing action on the liver. Known as cholagogues (the Greek word *khole* means bile), these plants trigger the liver's production of bile. As bile production is increased, the liver is gently cleansed. As toxins are cleared, the liver can focus on hormone function and the metabolism of fats and fatty acids, thus helping you maintain a healthy weight.

• **Dandelion root** (*Taraxacum officinale*) is completely nontoxic and gently restores liver function. It is rich in vitamins, minerals, and protein, and has more beta carotene and other carotenoids than carrots do. Dandelion enhances the flow of bile and is used in the treatment of liver congestion, hepatitis, gallstones, and jaundice. Dandelion also supports your kidneys. Dandelion can be taken by itself or in combination with other liver-support herbs.

Recommended dosage: 125 mg solid extract two or three times daily, or 30–50 mL root tincture two or three times daily, or 2–4 g powdered dried root two or three times daily. You can also buy dandelion in tea form. You can buy dandelion greens in some grocery stores; they make an excellent addition to salads.

• **Globe artichoke** (*Cynara scolymus*) has a long history of use in the treatment of many liver conditions. It has significant liver-protecting and liver-regenerating effects. Many digestive tonics contain artichoke. You can also eat artichokes to support liver health.

Recommended dosage: 500 mg three times daily, or eat the vegetable daily

• **Milk thistle** contains some of the most potent liver-protective substances known, including silymarin, which is a mixture of flavonoids, with silybin being the most active. Silymarin inhibits the action of free radicals (produced during normal body processes and as a result of external toxins), which damage liver cells. It also stimulates protein synthesis, which results in the production of new liver cells to replace the damaged ones. Milk thistle silymarin extract can help treat a wide range of liver disorders, including cirrhosis, viral hepatitis, and drug-induced disease. Silymarin enhances liver function to improve glucose control, important for managing weight. Most important, it stimulates the growth of new liver cells.

Recommended dosage: Take Milk thistle standardized to contain 80 percent silymarin; 50–100 mg per day.

• **Curcumin** (*Curcuma longa*), the yellow pigment of turmeric, has been used traditionally as a seasoning. Researchers have demonstrated that it has some very important healing benefits. Curcumin lowers the activity of cancer-causing agents while increasing their detoxification from the body. It is a potent antioxidant and a powerful liver detoxifier, and it acts as an anti-inflammatory. Curcumin also soothes the digestive tract.

Recommended dosage: 50–100 mg daily

• **Indole-3-carbinol** (I3C) is a plant nutrient found in broccoli, Brussels sprouts, cauliflower, and kale. It helps your body get rid of excess estrogen and environmental estrogens (xenoestrogens), as well as other toxic substances. I3C also inhibits the growth of prostate cancer, and reduces the development of tumors in the cervix and endometrium. Please note that for women with breast cancer, I3C is complementary and works alone and in combination with Tamoxifen™ (an estrogen-blocking drug for cancer) to inhibit the growth of estrogen-dominant cancers. Bodybuilders love I3C as it helps get rid of estrogen belly.

Recommended dosage: 150–300 mg daily

• **Calcium-D-glucarate** is found in fruits and vegetables such as apples, grapefruit, oranges, broccoli, and Brussels sprouts. It is a powerful antioxidant that increases the activity of other antioxidants such as vitamin C and carotenoids. Calcium-D-glucarate helps your body get rid of toxic substances through the liver; it prevents the estrogen couples from breaking up as they travel through the intestines and out of the body. Early research shows that it lowers the risk of breast, colon, prostate, lung, and liver cancers. Many of these cancers are also associated with obesity.

Recommended dosage: 150–300 mg daily

• **Lipoic acid** is a sulfur containing, vitamin-like substance. It plays an important role as a necessary cofactor in two vital energy-producing reactions involved in cellular energy. Lipoic acid is an effective antioxidant and acts on both water-soluble and fat-soluble free radicals. It aids detoxification of the liver. Lipoic acid has also been shown to prevent neuropathy and retinopathy in diabetics (see Chapter 9).

Recommended dosage: 100–300mg daily. For those with diabetic retinopathy or neuropathy, 600 mg daily

CONCLUSION

To ensure maximum weight loss and optimal health, you need to nourish your organs and correct imbalances. You will experience rapid and successful weight loss when you apply the principles learned in this chapter—and you will feel vibrant and full of energy.

chapter six

Weight-Loss Supplements

In earlier chapters I talked about what types of foods to eat to lose fat, how your emotions play a role in weight management, and how hormones can affect your increasing waist size. Certain natural compounds, along with the Body Sense eating plan and exercise program, can provide a kick-start to your weight-loss program. The bad news is that there are no magic pills or potions that will allow you to lose that weight overnight. But the good news is that science is finding many natural compounds to help enhance your metabolism or rev up your fat-burning furnace, promote lean muscle mass, prevent the storage of fat, suppress your appetite, support your thyroid, eliminate excess estrogens, and control cravings for food. If you have reduced your intake of calories, are exercising, and still can't lose weight—a syndrome called stubborn weight loss—there are supplements that will provide you with the extra push you need to start burning fat efficiently.

There is plenty of media and marketing hype regarding fat-loss products and much backlash from those who believe the claims should be halted and the products pulled from the shelves. But being overweight is killing people, increasing their rates of heart disease, diabetes, and cancer, and if a weight-loss product provides the incentive to keep people focused on a new eating plan or gives them the confidence to reach their goals, let them use these supplements to attain a healthy lifestyle.

In a perfect world you could obtain the nutrients you need from the food you eat, but today most people are eating the standard North American diet. For example, how many people eat the seven to ten half-cup (875–2500 mL) servings of fruits and vegetables they need just to get the minimum basic nutrients? Add to that exposure to environmental pollutants and too much stress, and people need even more vitamins, minerals, and other nutrients like essential fatty acids, enzymes, and coenzymes. In other words, there is not a single person in North America who can afford not to take nutritional supplements, especially a multivitamin with minerals and essential fatty acids (see Chapter 2). Don't take any of the supplements mentioned below without first ensuring you have a foundation of essential nutrients.

THERMOGENIC FAT-BURNING SUPPLEMENTS

Certain foods and supplements have the ability to increase your metabolic rate or burn fat more efficiently. They're called thermogenics because they rev up your metabolism. If you have been yo-yo dieting for years, you have taught your metabolism to slow down and conserve fat for later use. Thermogenic supplements will help reset your rate of metabolism.

FATS FOR FAT LOSS

Yes, eating fat can help you lose fat, but the fat you eat must be good fat (see Chapter 2). Restricting good fats from the diet has contributed to the massive numbers of overweight people. Several good fats—including conjugated linoleic acid (CLA), omega-3 fatty acids, and gamma linolenic acid (GLA)—have been found to improve weight loss.

Recent research shows that essential fatty acid (EFA) deficiency is related to low leptin levels. Leptin is a hormone that regulates appetite and brown fat thermogenesis; it also acts as a sensor of fat cell size. When a fat cell gets to a certain size, leptin signals the cell to eliminate fat. You can take EFA supplements to increase leptin levels, decrease appetite, and burn more fat. Mutations in the genes of leptin receptors are one possible cause of obesity.

Omega-6: GLA Aids Weight Loss

GLA, found primarily in the omega 6-oils from borage, evening primrose, and black currant, can help improve thyroid function, thus increasing metabolism and activating brown adipose tissue (BAT) to burn fat and correct genetic mutations in fat cells. BAT's job is to burn calories to increase body temperature and, when it functions correctly, it can be a powerful fat-burning furnace.

Omega-6 oils from canola, corn, sunflower, and safflower do not contain GLA. The body can convert these omega-6 oils to GLA and other fatty acids. However, many things can interfere with this conversion process, including stress, poor diet, lack of nutrients, and too many bad fats (saturated fats and trans-fatty acids) in the diet. I recommend borage oil and evening primrose oil as the most readily available and best sources of GLA for fat burning. Borage contains more GLA than evening primrose oil, hence the reason for differing dosages in the following recomendations.

Animal studies conducted by Dr. Takahashi from the National Food Research Institute in Ibaraki, Japan, have demonstrated that GLA also causes less body fat to accumulate. Dr. M.A. Mir, a researcher and consultant at the Welsh National School of Medicine in Cardiff, Wales, has shown that GLA from evening primrose oil and borage oil activates a metabolic process that can burn close to 50 percent of your body's total calories. In one study, by adding GLA, individuals lost between 9.6 and 11.4 lb. (4–5 kg) over a six-week period.

The late Dr. Horrobin, a professor of medicine at the University of Montreal, identified a calorie-burning mechanism that evening primrose oil helps regulate. The oil helps activate underactive brown fat in overweight people so they burn more calories. Dr. Horrobin described evening primrose oil as a safe, non-drug way to stimulate the body's metabolic activity and burn off fat.

More recently published studies have demonstrated the link between obesity and low GLA levels in lab animals. After supplementing with GLA, levels normalized, and the obese animals reduced their food intake, thus halting weight gain. Japanese research published in *The Journal of Nutrition* in 1994 confirmed that dietary GLA could reduce body fat by increasing brown fat activity, and that GLA may affect enzymes involved in the metabolism of fat and glucose.

Scientists believe that GLA, like other fatty acids, may have the potential to elevate levels of serotonin, a brain chemical that contributes to a feeling of fullness. Elevated serotonin levels would make you feel satisfied sooner; you would eat less and be less tempted to overindulge.

Your body also metabolizes GLA into hormone-like compounds (prostaglandins) that regulate a variety of actions in the body, including inflammation, muscle contraction, blood vessel dilation, and blood clotting. A deficiency of GLA can cause an imbalance between good prostaglandins and prostaglandins that promote inflammation (pain, redness, swelling and heat), which can lead to water retention and bloating. By supplementing with GLA, you can combat the hormonal water weight gain many women suffer.

Recommended dosage: Evening primrose oil, two 1000 mg capsules at breakfast and dinner; borage oil, one 1000 mg capsule at breakfast and dinner.

Omega-3: Fabulous Fat Burners

The omega-3 fatty acids (alpha-linolenic acid, ALA) are found primarily in flaxseed and fish and are associated with reduced fat storage, improvements in risk factors for heart disease and diabetes, skin conditions, immune function, and much more. Omega-3 fatty acids can be converted into eicosapentaenoic acid (EPA), docosahexaenoic acid (DHA), and prostaglandins. Fish oil supplements commonly contain 18 percent EPA and 12 percent DHA. The body must convert flaxseed oil to EPA and DHA and, depending on your ability to convert (most people using flaxseed oil only convert up to 11 percent to EPA and 5 percent to DHA), you may need both fish and flaxseed oils to get adequate EPA and DHA.

Recent research conducted by the Center for Human Nutrition at the University of Colorado Health Sciences Center examined the role of omega-3 fatty acids in improving metabolic fitness in moderately obese, hypertensive people. The study results showed that omega-3 fatty acids were effective in fat loss and also enhanced insulin sensitivity.

Omega-3 fatty acids increase the body's metabolic rate and thus help in fat burning. Ann Louise Gittleman, one of the premier nutritionists in the United States and author of *Eat Fat, Lose Weight* and *The Fat Flush Plan*, has seen tremendous weight loss in her clients who use flaxseed oil.

She recommends the addition of omega-3 oils to the diets of those who are suffering from obesity, diabetes, and high blood pressure.

Recommended dosage: 1–2 tbsp (15–30 mL) organic flaxseed oil or one to three 1,000 mg fish oil capsules from wild salmon, sardines, anchovies, and mackerel. (The smaller the fish, the fewer contaminants naturally found in the fish). Select a fish oil supplement that is pharmaceutical grade or molecularly distilled; such oils have been thoroughly checked to make sure they contain no harmful contaminants (PCBs or mercury).

CONJUGATED LINOLEIC ACID

Conjugated linoleic acid (CLA) is necessary for cell growth and as a building block of cell membranes. CLA occurs naturally in the meat and milk of cows that have been grass-fed; it is produced by the intestinal bacteria of these animals when they convert omega-6 linoleic acid into CLA. Humans cannot convert linoleic acid into CLA and must rely on food or supplements for CLA. Unfortunately, the CLA content of dairy and meat products has declined over the past few decades, due to changes in cattle food supplies from grass to grain, and to the increased use of antibiotics in cattle, which disrupt the gut flora in the cow, inhibiting the manufacture of CLA.

CLA is available as a convenient dietary supplement, made by converting the high linoleic acid content of either sunflower or safflower oils into CLA. To date there are more than 500 published research studies supporting CLA's ability to exert positive effects on fat loss, prevent and control Type 2 diabetes, protect against heart disease, reduce the risk of atherosclerosis, and regulate the immune response. CLA may also inhibit the growth of breast, prostate, and colon cancers.

More Muscle with CLA

Early animal research paved the way for groundbreaking work on CLA and fat loss in humans. The first human clinical trial using CLA was conducted in 1997 in Norway and published in *The Journal of Nutrition* in 2000. This study is, to date, the largest scientific evidence published showing CLA's effects on human fat tissue. The 90-day, double-blind, randomized, placebo-controlled study investigated the effects of different doses of CLA. Control groups receiving placebos were compared to subjects receiving 1.7–6.8 g of CLA per day. Results showed that 3.4 g of CLA per day was enough to obtain the fat-burning effects, and the group given the highest dose per day also experienced an increase in lean muscle mass. In fact, there was a remarkable 20 percent decrease in body fat, with an average loss of 7 lb. (3kg) of fat in the CLA group as compared to the placebo group. None of the subjects changed their diet. These results support previous observations that CLA is quite effective as a fat-fighting supplement and a producer of lean muscle mass.

CLA Keeps You Lean

In August 2000, a CLA researcher, Dr. Pariza, presented the long-awaited results of a clinical trial designed to assess the effects of CLA on the body composition of obese men and women. Eighty overweight people took part in the six-month study in which they dieted and exercised. As expected, most initially lost weight, but once their diets ended, many regained some of their weight. The participants who were not given CLA put the pounds back on predominantly as fat, whereas those who took CLA regularly regained less fat and retained more muscle mass. The results also showed that CLA made it easier for the participants to stay on their diets.

CLA and Exercise

The next logical question for those studying CLA would be: Does CLA influence the effects of exercise? A Norwegian study published in 2001 in *The Journal of International Medical Research* says that it does. This double-blind, randomized, placebo-controlled trial focused on twenty healthy volunteers recruited from a physical fitness center. For the trial, they trained for ninety minutes of strenuous exercise, three times a week. The volunteers did not make any changes to their lifestyle or diet during this trial. The study shows that those participants who ingested 1.8 g of CLA per day for twelve weeks experienced significant body fat reduction compared to the control group. The control group continued to exercise but received a placebo instead of CLA. Again, CLA reduced body fat, but because the lean muscle mass was increased, there was no change in actual body weight.

Recommended dosage: 4,000–6,000 mg per day in a divided dose at breakfast and dinner.

CITRUS AURANTIUM

Long used in traditional Chinese medicine, *Citrus aurantium* is the immature dried fruit of the bitter orange. A natural stimulant, *Citrus aurantium* supplies synephrine, which is a thermogenic known to increase resting metabolism rate, thus helping the body burn fat more efficiently. *Citrus aurantium* also improves energy levels, especially during aerobic exercise, allowing you to work out longer and with more endurance.

Citrus aurantium contains five active ingredients that resemble adrenaline's physiological actions. Of the five, synephrine is the best known and most studied constituent. Synephrine is as effective as ephedra without the negative side effects. Ephedra, another well-known weight loss ingredient, boosts metabolism and suppresses appetite, but is also known to negatively stimulate the cardiovascular system, increasing heart rate and blood pressure, and can promote heart palpitations, seizures, stroke, nervousness, insomnia, and anxiety. Synephrine does not do this.

Synephrine binds to certain receptor sites on fat cells to stimulate fat burning and fat mobilization and has been shown to safely enhance fat loss. Synephrine has also been shown to reduce appetite and provide a subtle energy boost to users. Synephrine is found in all citrus fruits.

Recommended dosage: *Citrus aurantium*, bitter orange extract with 6 percent synephrine, 150–325 mg per day.

YERBA MATÉ EXTRACT

Natural sources of caffeine, in low doses, are effective in aiding weight loss. When taken with synephrine, caffeine amplifies synephrine's thermogenic effects. Yerba maté is a natural form of caffeine. The dosage recommended below contains less than the equivalent of one-eighth of a cup of coffee per serving. Yerba maté is a stimulant used to reduce food cravings. Traditionally yerba maté has been used to balance blood sugar levels, and modern research suggests it may be useful in treating diabetes. Overweight people are at higher risk for cellular damage and thus an increased risk for heart disease, cancer, and diabetes. Yerba maté is a valued antioxidant that destroys the substances that cause cellular damage.

Recommended dosage: 200 mg per day.

GREEN TEA EXTRACT

Did you know that sipping that cup of green tea or swallowing that green tea tablet can help fight cancer, prevent gum disease, slow the aging process, and aid fat loss? Thousands of research studies have confirmed the beneficial effects of green tea. According to Michael Murray, N.D., in his new book, *How to Prevent and Treat Cancer with Natural Medicine*, "Both green and black tea are derived from the same plant *Camelia sinensis*. Of the nearly 2.5 million tons of dried tea produced each year, only 20 percent is green tea." Green tea, as science has confirmed, is the healthier choice as it contains compounds called polyphenols, which are known for their powerful healing effects.

The manufacturing process is what makes the difference between green and black tea. Green tea is produced by lightly steaming the fresh-cut leaf, so it is not fermented and provides high levels of polyphenols. Oolong tea is partially fermented, and black tea is fully fermented. During the fermentation process, enzymes convert the polyphenols to compounds with much less activity.

Research has been conducted into green tea's fat-burning properties. A small study revealed that participants who took three green tea extract capsules daily increased their fat burning without accelerating their heart rate. The capsules safely melted fat away. Caffeine effectively enhances the fat-burning effects of the synephrine, thus improving fat loss.

Soothes the Flames of Inflammation

Several recent studies showed that green tea reduced pain and swelling in people with arthritis. Green tea was found to be as effective as some anti-inflammatory medications such as Celebrex™. Green tea also contains fifty-one other anti-inflammatory compounds. The USDA Phytochemical Database also identified fifteen anti-ulcer compounds in green tea, supporting evidence that long-term use can inhibit ulcers caused by prolonged use of nonsteroidal anti-inflammatory medications, including ibuprofen. With reduced inflammation, your exercise routines will become effortless. Inflammation is a process where our immune system sends factors out to heal an injury or kill an invader. It also affects our fat cell membranes and hormone function, making them resistant to weight loss. Herbs and nutrients that reduce inflammation improve weight management, as well.

Green Tea and Blood Sugar

To prevent or treat diabetes, you can either enhance insulin function, which helps control blood sugar levels, or suppress blood sugar levels through other means, such as diet (see Chapter 9). In the USDA tea study, humans in clinical trials took 200–500 mg of green tea in capsule or tablet form before ingesting starch. Starch gets converted to glucose by digestive enzymes. But in the study, glucose production was inhibited, and the uptake of glucose by the intestine to the bloodstream was suppressed. Those studying the anti-obesity effects of green tea believe this is the reason for green tea's fat-loss benefits.

Calming the Caffeine Kick

Worried about getting too much caffeine from green tea? Drinking 3 cups (750 mL) provides about the same amount of caffeine as 1 cup (250 mL) of drip coffee. Green tea also contains L-theanine, which negates side effects of caffeine such as hypertension and sleep disturbances. L-theanine is very well researched and has been shown to promote relaxation without drowsiness, improve learning and concentration, support immune function, lower cholesterol, and reduce stress and anxiety. Now you know why you can drink several cups of green tea and not develop the caffeine jitters.

Recommended dosage: 200 mg per day of green tea extract. Supplement the fat-burning effects of green tea capsules by drinking green tea as well.

CAYENNE PEPPER

Several clinical studies have shown that cayenne pepper increases thermogenesis. Capsicum, the active ingredient in cayenne pepper, when used in combination with other thermogenic agents, including green tea and bitter orange, enhances metabolism and energy.

Recommended dosage: 100 mg per day.

GINGER ROOT

Ginger root improves digestion and, when used in combination with other herbs, enhances metabolism and reduces food cravings.

Recommended dosage: 50 mg per day. Ginger tea is also an excellent alternative to coffee.

5-HTP (5-HYDROXYTRYPTOPHAN)

Another important nutrient in weight loss is 5-hydroxytryptophan, commonly called 5-HTP, which is a breakdown product of the amino acid tryptophan. Proteins in the food we eat provide you with amino acids, one of which is tryptophan. Tryptophan is broken down by vitamins and enzymes into 5-HTP, which is turned into serotonin, the neurotransmitter that tells your brain you are satisfied and do not need to eat any more. Serotonin deficiency contributes to carbohydrate cravings (sugar cravings), overeating, and obesity. A healthy liver is essential to proper conversion of tryptophan to 5-HTP and then into serotonin. You also need adequate levels of magnesium, vitamin B6, niacin (vitamin B3), and proper insulin function. Insulin resistance inhibits the conversion of 5-HTP. 5-HTP reduces appetite, enhances your mood, increases your energy levels, and controls sugar cravings. 5-HTP has also been extensively researched for the treatment of depression, as well as insomnia and other sleep disorders.

5-HTP occurs naturally in the seeds of *Griffonia simplicifolia* and is extracted from that plant and put into capsules. Look for pharmaceutical grade 5-HTP in enteric-coated capsules for optimal results.

Recommended dosage: 50–100 mg three times per day at breakfast, dinner, and before bed. If you have not noticed an improvement in mood or a reduction in cravings after four weeks, increase to 200 mg three times per day.

Note: If you are taking MAO inhibitors or antidepressants, do *not* take 5-HTP at the same time.

PHASEOLAMIN 2250 (PHASE 2)

Phase 2™ is a standardized extract derived from the white kidney bean that promotes weight loss by neutralizing ingested starches. In clinical studies Phase 2 has been shown to reduce blood sugar after starchy meals and promote loss of body fat. Specifically, it works in the intestine by temporarily inhibiting the activity of the enzyme alpha-amylase, which converts starch into glucose; with Phase 2, fewer starch calories are absorbed from food.

A test-tube study found that Phase 2 neutralized 2,250 starch calories, or the equivalent of more than 1 lb. (.5 kg) of spaghetti or one loaf of bread. Preliminary human studies have confirmed this effect. In another study, starch absorption averaged 57 percent less in subjects taking Phase 2 than in those taking a placebo. After-meal glucose levels were measured as an index of starch absorption. After an overnight fast, glucose levels were measured and participants were then randomized to receive a standard-ized meal containing 60 g (2 oz) starch (equivalent to four slices of bread) and either a placebo or 1,500 mg of Phase 2. Participants went about their regular activities, and glucose was measured every twenty minutes for four hours after the meal.

Participants receiving Phase 2 in another study averaged an 85 percent reduction in glucose response. In this study, all parameters were the same as the study above with the exception that test subjects were inactive dur-ing the course of the day. This study was undertaken to determine whether differences in physical activity affected the outcome. The results of these two studies strongly indicate that most of the starch calories from the test meal were undigested when taken with Phase 2. Participants given Phase 2 noted no side effects.

An extensive double-blind, placebo-controlled study involving sixty healthy men and women aged twenty-five to forty-five used only Phase 2. Participants were instructed to follow a recommended diet with daily con-sumption of starchy foods (potatoes, pasta) during one of the principal meals. Participants who consumed 500 mg of Phase 2 once daily before the starchy meal lost an average of 6.45 lb. (3 kg) by the end of the thirty-day study; those consuming a placebo lost an average of 0.76 lb. (0.5 kg). In addition, those on Phase 2 lost 10.45 percent of fat and 3.44 percent of their waist circumference. These losses occurred without any change in lean muscle mass. We do not want to lose muscle when we are dieting, because muscle helps burn fat.

The carbohydrate-neutralizing effect of Phase 2 is a novel approach to weight loss and may be particularly helpful for those struggling with obe-sity and diabetes. Phase 2 is safe and well tolerated and is not known to interact with any drugs or supplements. Phase 2 will soon be added to many common foods to help deal with obesity in North America.

Recommended dosage: 500 mg once or twice a day before starch-rich meals.

CASSIA NOMAME EXTRACT

Cassia nomame, a member of the cinnamon family, is a lipase inhibitor. Lipase is the enzyme that digests fat, so by blocking lipase, *Cassia nomame* significantly reduces the amount of fat absorbed by your body by about 30 percent. Research in Japan suggests it could be used for the prevention and/or treatment of obesity. Combined with Phase 2, this herb provides even better results.

Recommended dosage: 75 mg per day.

GYMNEMA SYLVESTRE EXTRACT

Gymnema sylvestre, a plant native to India and used in traditional medicine, contains special plant-sugar compounds referred to as gymnemic acid. Gymnema extract seems to improve the action of insulin and reduce fasting blood sugar levels, and it improves overall blood sugar control. Gymnema does not lower blood sugar or cause hypoglycemic effects in healthy individuals. It will, however, reduce the absorption of sugar and reduce cholesterol. Gymnema is effective at controlling appetite. Weight loss can be improved by maintaining healthy, stable blood sugar levels.

Recommended dosage: 50 mg per day.

GARCINIA CAMBOGIA (HYDROXYCITRIC)

Garcinia cambogia, a fruit from India, contains hydroxycitric acid (HCA), a potent fat-burning chemical. HCA helps halt the conversion of carbohydrates into fat and increases fat-releasing enzymes that cause fat to be released from fat cells and burned in the body as fuel. It also inhibits excess glucose-stimulated insulin secretion. HCA is available in a form bound to magnesium, making it a more effective fat burner.

Recommended dosage: 500–2,000 mg per day. *Garcinia cambogia* is also available in a tea. Use the tea as an alternative to caffeinated beverages and watch your weight melt off.

IODINE AND THYROID HEALTH

Normalizing the function of thyroid gland is essential for weight management. Low thyroid hormones (hypothyroidism) cause weight gain, slow metabolism, hormone dysfunction, hair loss, and sensitivity to heat or cold (see Chapter 4). The thyroid gland needs iodine to make its hormones. Too little iodine in the diet can impair thyroid function, while too much can overstimulate and impair the thyroid's ability to make hormones.

Recommended dosage: 200–400 mcg per day, or 1 mcg per 2.2 lb. (1 kg) body weight. People with overactive thyroid function (hyperthyroidism) should avoid excess iodine.

PROTEIN POWDERS

The importance of protein for optimal health cannot be overstated. Protein is made up of twenty amino acids. Twelve of these are synthesized by the liver, and the remaining eight, which are called "essential," must be obtained from food. The richest sources of amino acids include legumes, fresh fish, free-range poultry, free-range eggs, nuts, seeds, fermented soy, whey protein, and fermented dairy products. Protein powder is an essential food in the Body Sense Natural Diet program. It is quick, delicious, and you don't have to cook it. Many diseases are related to inadequate protein consumption in the diet, especially:

- osteoporosis
- a weak immune system
- fragile, soft nails
- thinning hair
- wrinkled skin
- lack of muscle tone, sagging chin
- breast cancer
- hormonal dysfunction
- heart problems
- poor healing of wounds
- increased aging
- hypoglycemia
- poor digestion
- depression due to a lack of serotonin
- incontinence

FAT BURNING BREAKFAST

Did you know that by eating a protein-rich breakfast you can increase your body's ability to burn fat by 25 percent, and that the fat-burning action will last all day? Carbohydrate-rich breakfast cereals, skim milk, and toast slow your fat-burning rate, keep you feeling hungry, and increase your food cravings. Worse yet, when you skip meals, your metabolic rate slows to conserve energy because you are starving your body. Then when you do eat, the calories are stored as fat. The answer is to eat breakfast every day, along with several small meals throughout the day. Drink a protein-rich shake every morning for breakfast and again as a snack in the afternoon to ensure that your body feels satisfied and your fat-burning furnace is working at peak levels.

How Much Protein Do You Need?

Adult men	70 g
Adult women	58 g
Pregnant women	65 g
Lactating women	75 g
Girls aged 13–15	62 g
Girls aged 16–20	58 g
Boys aged 13–15	75 g
Boys aged 16–20	85 g

Recommended dosage: One or two scoops of whey protein powder will provide up to 20 g protein. Two rounded tablespoons of fermented soy powder provide approximately 11 g protein. One egg provides 7 g protein. One ounce (30 g) meat, fish, or cheese will provide 7 g protein. Four ounces (113 g) of tofu provides 7 g protein. Vary your sources of protein and include two shakes per day, one for breakfast and one in the afternoon. For optimal weight loss, the Body Sense eating plan contains about 60 g protein per day.

Biological Value of Dietary Proteins

Protein	*Biological Value*
Lactalbumin (found in whey protein concentrate)	104
Whole egg	100
Cow's milk	91
Egg whites	88
Fish	83
Beef	80
Chicken	79
Casein	77
Soy	74
Rice	59
Beans, seeds, nuts	49

The higher the biological value (BV) of protein, the more complete the protein is, meaning the more essential amino acids it contains. Mother's milk is the perfect protein, and the next best protein is the egg, against which all other proteins are measured.

Some people have greater protein requirements than others. If you are very active, exercise strenuously, do heavy labor, or are pregnant, you will need more protein than if you are a couch potato. On average, you should make protein 15–20 percent of your diet. When choosing your protein sources, opt for free-range poultry and eggs and wild fish over farm-grown to avoid contamination from antibiotics and growth hormones. Purchase nuts in the shell and buy organic legumes. If you need to keep your glucose levels stable, split your protein requirements into three or four small portions and eat them spaced throughout the day. Women rarely get enough protein because of their food choices and calorie restrictive diets.

WHEY PROTEIN AND FAT-BURNING PROTEIN

Whey protein contains alpha-lactalbumin, glycomacropeptides, lactoferrin, and amino acids, including tryptophan and glutathione precursors. Each component in whey protein has a unique action. When all the components are combined, they have powerful healing capabilities:

• Alpha-lactalbumin in whey protein is the key to the manufacture of protein in your body. Its consumption enhances tryptophan and immune function and reduces the stress hormone cortisol, which causes your fat cells to become resistant to fat loss.
• Tryptophan, used by the brain to manufacture serotonin, is a key neurotransmitter. A tryptophan deficiency can lead to depression, anxiety, moodiness, and insomnia. People who lack serotonin generally eat more.
• Glutathione, the most powerful detoxifier in your body, is integral to a healthy immune system. It is an antiviral, fights cancer, protects you against free radicals, and extends life. It is also important for a healthy liver.
• Glycomacropeptides stimulate the pancreatic hormone cholecystokinin (CCK), which is responsible for the release of enzymes from the pancreas and for the contraction of the gallbladder and the bowels. It is also responsible for telling your brain you are satisfied and no longer require more food, so it helps control your appetite.

• Lactoferrin, an antioxidant, is a powerful antiviral and antibacterial agent shown to inhibit the growth of *E. coli*, salmonella, and *Candida* in the gut. It also helps ensure the optimal use of iron in the body by binding to iron and preventing its oxidation.

PROTEIN PROTECTS YOUR HEART

We have all heard that often the first sign of a heart attack is death. Heart disease is the number one killer of North Americans and protein may be a powerful treatment in the battle against heart disease. Protein is essential to a healthy heart as it keeps our insulin levels stable. The American Diabetes Association has always recommended that we eat more protein (30% of the diet should be protein) and fewer carbohydrates to keep our insulin normalized. What does insulin have to do with heart disease? High insulin causes certain enzymes to convert lipids in our bloodstream into heart and artery damaging substances. This is why diabetics are prone to cardiovascular disease. Small protein meals throughout the day have been recommended for diabetics and those with hypoglycemia (low blood sugar) as an effective measure in the treatment and prevention of heart disease and to maintain healthy insulin levels.

LOWER CHOLESTEROL AND TRIGLYCERIDES

Results from more than fifty studies have provided scientific evidence of the cholesterol-lowering benefits of soy protein in the diet. Twenty-five to fifty grams of isolated soy protein will effectively lower total cholesterol and LDL, the bad cholesterol, while maintaining HDL, the good cholesterol. So effective is soy protein at lowering cholesterol and triglycerides and preventing narrowing of the arteries that the U.S. Food and Drug Association has allowed a health claim that states, "soy may protect against the development of coronary heart disease." Coronary heart disease, which causes more than 500,000 deaths per year from heart attack, is characterized by obstruction in the arteries and other blood vessels.

PROTEIN SHAKES

A protein shake containing whey and fermented soy provides low-calorie protein that will enhance your fat-burning furnace. Whey protein contains the hormone CCK, which makes you feel full and satisfied, thereby reducing food cravings. Fermented soy powder was recently studied at Beth Israel Medical Center in Boston for its effects in promoting weight loss in obese animals. Animals fed fermented soy powder lost as much as 64 percent of their body fat. As well, they did not eat as much food as the animals who didn't get fermented soy powders, providing evidence that food cravings were reduced.

Protein shakes are refreshing, provide quick energy, and are a wonderful alternative to caffeine-laden beverages. Excess consumption of caffeine can lead to a magnesium deficiency resulting in heart palpitations, twitchy eyelids, high blood pressure, anxiety, sleep disturbances, stress, osteoporosis, restless legs, urinary tract infections, and fibroid breast cysts.

SOY PROTEIN

Soy protein is also rich in many plant nutrients, including sterols and sterolins, inositol hexaphosphate, saponins, genistein, daidzein, lignans, and protease inhibitors. Soy is an alternative source of protein for vegetarians who do not want to consume whey or animal proteins. Soy must be eaten fermented along with a varied diet rich in fruits, vegetables, sea vegetables (like kelp), nuts, and seeds.

The isoflavones genistein and daidzein, abundantly found in soy, act as anticancer agents that may reverse or retard the cancer process. Studies show that genistein interferes with angiogenesis, a process cancer cells use to grow new blood vessels and thus ensure their survival. By halting the production of new blood vessels, genistein starves the cancer. Genistein has also been shown to induce programmed cell death (apoptosis) in cancer cells. As well, genistein binds to estrogen receptors and blocks some of estrogen's detrimental effects, which promote the growth of cancer. In studies, daidzein increased T-cells (which help fight viruses, bacteria, and cancer) and macrophage (the big eating cells of the immune system) activity, both important for strengthening immunity. Genistein and daidzein are predominantly sold for their ability to reduce hot flashes and night sweats in menopausal women.

The protease inhibitors in soy counteract the effects of cancer-causing fatty acids and prevent the activation of specific genes that can cause cancer. Protease inhibitors also protect against the effects of radiation and free radicals, which damage our DNA.

There is much human research on the ability of sterols and sterolins to regulate immune function, thus reducing allergic reactions, controlling inflammation, treating viral infections, and generally improving overall immune function. Large doses of sterols alone have been found to be very effective at lowering cholesterol, thereby reducing the risk of heart disease.

Phytates, long viewed as a detrimental component of soy because they can bind to minerals and inhibit the production of thyroid hormones, are now thought to be helpful because they can bind iron in the intestines. Unbound iron generates harmful free radicals, which are thought to be a precursor to cancer. Excess iron has also been associated with heart disease.

Soy is also very high in plant lignans, which are converted in the colon by bacterial fermentation. Lignans are structurally similar to estrogens and work as weak estrogens or anti-estrogens: they remove excess estrogens that may be harmful or cancer promoting. Lignans have also been shown to balance estrogen metabolism in women and men. And lignans are antibacterial, antifungal, and antiviral. Excellent research has shown that lignans effectively reduce the risk of breast cancer in women and reduce tumor size in women with breast cancer

Women are not the only ones to benefit from soy. Men who consume one or two servings of soy beverage per day are 70 percent less likely to develop prostate cancer than men who drink cow's milk.

To be on the safe side, women with estrogen receptor-positive breast cancers should avoid soy foods. Although research has not shown an increase in breast cancer growth in women consuming soy who have estrogen receptor-positive breast cancer due to the weak estrogenic activity of soy, it is suggested that women with this type of cancer avoid it to be on the safe side.

Whey and fermented soy protein also keep your blood sugar levels stabilized. Healthy blood sugar levels are key to reducing body fat. When you eat carbohydrate-laden meals (white sugar, white flour, white rice, white potatoes, breakfast cereals, white pasta), you also dramatically increase your blood sugar and subsequent release of insulin. When insulin is too high it increases your risk of heart disease, diabetes, and obesity. If when blood sugar is too low (hypoglycemia) from not eating enough protein, you will experience mood swings, feel lethargic and weak, and crave food. The Canadian and American Diabetes

Associations recommend that 30 percent of the diet should be from protein sources. You can maintain healthy insulin levels by eating small protein meals throughout the day.

Build Stronger Bones and Get Healthier Nails, Hair, and Skin

Soy and whey protein are both important foods in the prevention and treatment of osteoporosis. Soy in particular has been shown to increase bone density and bone mineral content in the lumbar spine. Researchers also believe that soy may also inhibit bone breakdown. Studies show that soy prevents bone loss in rats that had their ovaries removed. The body needs adequate estrogen to keep bones strong. In one study researchers compared genistein to steroidal estrogen. They found that 1 mg per day of genistein was equivalent to 5 mcg per day of steroidal estrogens in maintaining bone mass. Isoflavones in soy act as weak estrogens, supplying the estrogen needed to prevent bone loss and improve bone density. Two human studies using soy protein found significant increases in the bone-mineral content of the lumbar spine, and in general bone-mineral density.

Whey protein has also been researched for its ability to promote bone formation. Whey protein activates osteoblasts, the cells that form bone, and also increases total protein and collagen. Whey protein combined with soy should be part of your program to treat or prevent osteoporosis. Another excellent benefit of soy and whey is that they are relatively high in calcium and magnesium, both important for bone health.

Protein and collagen are the ingredients that make strong nails and gorgeous thick, shiny, hair. Protein keeps your muscles from sagging and prevents double chins and wrinkled skin. Strong muscles help you burn fat more efficiently, keep you younger looking, and provide strength for a beautiful body.

Why Fermented Soy Instead of Regular Soy?

There has been much controversy regarding soy's health benefits over the past few years. North Americans are consuming more soy because of heavy marketing and promotion and the misinterpreted research that evaluated the reduced rates of heart disease, cancer, osteoporosis, and menopause symptoms in Asian countries. Scientists believed the reduced rates of these conditions were due mainly to the soy foods that people in those countries eat. Asian diets contain fermented soy in the form of tempeh, miso, and soy sauce, which is a completely different type of soy food compared to regular non-fermented soybeans.In North America all the soy sold is derived from Genetically Modified organisms (GMO) to be sprayed with more of the herbicide Round-up™ so that the plant will not die from repeated or heavy applications of Round-up. It is called Round-up-ready soy. Unless it is cleary marked as organic, it is GMO soy. GMO foods are very controversial as they have not been extensively studied in a human population—we are currently the experiment for these foods. We should avoid GM foods at all cost. Look for organic fermented soy products to be on the safe side.

LIVER AND HORMONE HELPING SUPPLEMENTS

Your liver is the organ in which proteins and carbohydrates are metabolized, hormones are processed and transported for uses elsewhere in the body, toxins are dealt with, and fats and cholesterol are digested and assimilated (see Chapter 3). Optimal performance is crucial if you want to maintain your ideal weight. The following nutrients are important, especially for women who have hormone-induced weight gain or excess fat around the middle. Many of them help balance your hormones and detoxify excess estrogens, which make both men and women fat around the abdominal area.

Indole-3-Carbinol

Indole-3-carbinol (I3C) is one of my favorite nutrients. It is an anti-cancer plant nutrient found in cruciferous vegetables such as broccoli, Brussels sprouts, cauliflower, kale, and cabbage. Research has shown that I3C helps to break down cancer-causing estrogens to non-toxic forms, and it eliminates harmful estrogen mimickers found in pesticides, plastics, cosmetics, and more. I3C improves the detoxification of excess estrogen or xenoestrogens. Indole-3-carbinol also increases the conversion of cancer-causing estrogens and dangerous estrogens produced by the body to non-toxic estrogens, so it protects against hormone-dominant cancers, i.e.. breast, prostate, and ovarian. It also reduces tumour development in the endometrium and cervix. As you can see, this potent nutrient is essential in balancing hormones for proper fat management. Both men and women, but especially women over forty, have been telling their friends and fitness trainers that their hormones must be making them fat because they exercise and cut back on calories, but still do not lose weight. Indole-3-carbinol improves hormone balance in the liver, ensuring that your estrogens don't make you fat and it improves the ratio of estrogen to progesterone and testosterone. Watch the estrogen belly melt away with this super nutrient.

Recommended dosage: 150–300 mg per day.

Calcium-D-glucarate

Calcium-D-glucarate is found in all fruits and vegetables, with the highest concentrations in apples, grapefruit, and broccoli. In addition to benefits in cancer prevention, calcium-D-glucarate has been shown to reduce total triglyceride levels by an average of 12 percent, hence reducing the risk of cardiovascular disease. It also helps rid the body of toxic substances by way of the liver, where dangerous substances are combined to be safely excreted from the body. Calcium-D-glucarate removes excess estrogens and xenoestrogens. It also inhibits tumour formation caused by cancer-causing chemical agents. Calcium-D-glucarate is a powerful detoxifier of excess estrogens via the liver, another fabulous fat-flushing nutrient.

Recommended dosage: 150–300 mg per day.

Curcumin (Turmeric)

Curcumin is the yellow pigment of turmeric, the chief ingredient in curry. It is a powerful anti-inflammatory agent and inhibits all steps of cancer development. Curcumin also helps to eliminate cancer-causing estrogens and environmental estrogens via the liver, and supports the liver in all its functions. Curcumin lowers the activity of carcinogens while increasing detoxification and enhancing glutathione, the most powerful detoxifier of the liver. Most importantly for fat loss, it helps the liver detoxify xenoestrogens, pesticides, and residues of prescription medications. All of these substances congest the liver, promoting fatty liver.

Recommended dosage: 50–100 mg per day. Ensure that your curcumin supplement contains 95 percent curcumin.

Milk Thistle

Milk thistle is the most common liver-supporting nutrient that enhances detoxification of excess and toxic estrogens from the liver. Milk thistle is called the protector of the liver and helps to stimulate the growth of healthy new liver cells and promote bile flow. Milk thistle improves estrogen balance by ensuring that estrogen stays in its healthy form. Milk thistle also increases intracellular glutathione production by 35 percent in healthy people, providing protection from toxins and reducing the aging process.

Recommended dosage: 50–100 mg per day, Milk thistle should be at least 80 percent silymarin.

L-Carnitine

L-carnitine, found mainly in lean beef and lamb and made primarily in the liver, plays a vital role in metabolizing fatty acids. It is also concentrated in human breast milk and colostrum (first milk). L-carnitine carries fatty acids into the mitochondria (the powerhouse of the cell), where it is changed into energy. In simpler terms, L-carnitine assists the mitochondria in burning fat as fuel. L-carnitine also helps eliminate wastes from the mitochondria, ensuring optimal functioning of this important organelle. It also aids in disorders of the mitochondria, such as chronic fatigue syndrome and muscular conditions. L-carnitine can help you lose that fatty layer around your abdomen.

Recommended dosage: 1 g of L-carnitine on an empty stomach per day. L-carnitine is readily available in the United States, but not in Canada. Health Canada regulations may change in 2005. Canadians can order L-carnitine over the Internet and import one or two bottles per month for personal use.

Chromium

Chromium used to be found in abundance in whole grains, but overfarming has depleted our soils of chromium, leading to a prevalence of chromium deficiency in North Americans. Chromium, a trace mineral, is key to maintaining insulin stability, stimulates the manufacture of fatty acids and cholesterol, activates digestive enzymes, and protects our RNA and DNA. High blood sugar levels cause a corresponding spike in insulin, which leads to weight gain. Because of its influence on insulin and its suppression of sugar cravings, chromium is important for those with Type 2 diabetes, hypoglycemia (low blood sugar), and both weight loss and gain. It also lowers triglycerides and blood cholesterol levels. Deficiency of chromium leads to glucose intolerance and atherosclerosis (hardening of the arteries). Chromium reduces the cells' resistance to insulin, meaning that your cells won't let insulin into the cell so that too much insulin remains in the blood, promoting insulin resistance, Syndrome X, diabetes, and weight gain.

Recommended dosage: 200–400 mcg per day.

CONCLUSION

The next obvious question is, "Do I need all these supplements?" No, not all, but you do need essential fatty acids, protein, and a multivitamin with minerals, including chromium every day. If you have been dieting for years, try some of the thermogenics I mentioned, along with protein powder, for forty-two days and watch your new body emerge. Thermogenics will give you a boost of energy just before you do your morning workout or clean the house. If you just have to have a bowl of pasta or some potatoes, use the starch blocker. Some of the nutrients I recommend will have amazing effects on your moods, a nice benefit along with the fat burning action. Remember, you must take a multivitamin with minerals and essential fatty acids. All the other nutrients are optional. You will want to read Chapter 9 if you have diabetes because diabetics need different supplements to regulate blood sugar for managing weight loss. If you decide not to take any of the thermogenics or nutrients, you will successfully lose weight if you follow the diet and exercise recommendations and correct your hormone imbalances. Fat loss supplements add a little boost to your program, so you get results quickly. People who have followed the Body Sense plan for several years swear by the thermogenics, protein powders and 5-HTP, which maximize and speed up weight loss over the six-week program.

Fast, Fun Fitness

Less than twenty five percent of North American adults exercise regularly. In an attempt to cut costs, some schools have discontinued sports activities and decreased the hours spent per week in physical education classes. Children and adults are spending more time performing sedentary tasks like surfing the Internet, playing video games, and watching television. This lack of exercise adds to insulin resistance, hormone dysfunction, and inevitable weight gain. Your body is designed to move. The adage "Move it or lose it" is true when it comes to your muscles. Remember that the more muscles you have, the more fat you burn. Your muscles are full of tiny engines (called mitochondria) that need plenty of fuel, which they get from fat. By simply adding 5 lb. (2 kg) of nice, lean muscles, you will burn an additional 250 calories per day, or 25 lb. (11.5 kg) of fat per year.

Studies in Finland demonstrated that exercising for a little longer than half an hour four times a week or forty-five minutes three times a week reduces your risk of heart attack by fifty percent and stroke by forty percent.

By performing the exercises described in this chapter, you will lose on average 1–2 lb. (0.5–1 kg) per week. The Body Sense Natural Diet will help you burn about 65–75 percent of fat while building lean muscles. Many women are worried that exercise will build muscles and they will end up looking like Arnold Schwarzenegger. Don't worry. The Body Sense program builds sexy, beautiful arms that won't have that jiggling, hanging skin between your armpit and your elbow, your chin line will stop sagging, your thighs will stop slapping together, cellulite will diminish, and wait until you see what happens to your breasts and stomach. Another benefit of muscle is that it helps you burn calories even while you are sleeping or sitting in your chair.

SLOW AGING AND LIVE LONGER

Mental clarity, more strength and stamina, normal blood sugar, reversal of syndrome X, and improved cardiovascular health will not only improve your overall health but ensure that you live longer too. Within six weeks the Body Sense Natural Diet program provides these benefits.

We could call the Body Sense program the fountain of youth. Now that you are taking nutritional supplements every day, eating a healthy diet, and exercising ten minutes per day, you will notice that your skin is glowing and firmer, your hair thicker, your muscles stronger, and you will have a spring in your step, just like when you were younger.

According to the American College of Sports Medicine, approximately 250,000 deaths a year in the United States are related to lack of physical activity, which promotes heart disease, diabetes, cancer, and obesity.

You are never too old or too unfit to begin an exercise program; in fact, being unfit is all the more reason to start. Study after study has come to the same conclusion: inactivity promotes illness, and the right exercise for the condition can work wonders in reversing or delaying that illness. Activity encourages the flow of oxygen and other nutrients and enhances mood. An article published in *Diabetes Care* by Japanese researchers confirmed that exercise lowers triglycerides, improves insulin sensitivity, and stabilizes glucose tolerance in Type 2 adult-onset diabetics.

Diseases related to excess weight:

- Early death
- Type 2 diabetes
- Insulin resistance
- Obesity
- High blood pressure

- High cholesterol and triglycerides
- Stroke
- Osteoarthritis (an extra 10 lb./4.5 kg causes an additional 40 lb./18 kg of extra pressure on the hips, knees, and ankles)
- Osteoporosis
- Gout
- Cancers of all types (especially breast, colon, and endometrial cancer)
- Kidney disease
- Accelerated aging
- Depression
- Weak immune system
- Pain and inflammation
- Extreme menopause symptoms

Have no fear. Weight loss can reverse these conditions.

Exercise Program

Start with the ten-minute weight-bearing exercise program every morning. Exercising in the morning revs up your metabolic rate, which aids calorie burning throughout the day. When you exercise, your cortisol levels naturally rise. Avoid evening exercise if possible, as high nighttime cortisol levels can disrupt sleep and add stress to the body.

Combine the Body Sense ten-minute weight-bearing exercise program with walking, gardening, dancing, even cleaning your house—and move vigorously to burn excess fat. Science tells you that exercise improves your cardiovascular system and helps reverse the signs of aging. When your skin is taut, you don't look as old. Regular exercise also helps you move faster. You will be sure of yourself, and you will feel strong.

Calories Burned by Physical Activity

These are the calories expended by a 125 lb. (57 kg) woman doing ten minutes of the following activities:

Activity	Calories Expended
Making beds	32
Weeding	49

House painting	29
Dancing	35
Swimming (front crawl)	40
Tennis	56
Walking (briskly)	52
Walking (leisurely stroll)	29
Running	90
Cycling	42
Cross-country skiing	98
Downhill skiing	80
Shoveling snow	65

(*Source*: John Foreyt, Ph. D., Baylor College of Medicine's Behavior Medicine Research Center; Kelly D. Brownell, Ph.D., Yale University; and Thomas A. Wadden, Ph.D., University of Pennsylvania School of Medicine)

Effortless Exercise

Before you begin, go to a fitness store or the fitness section of your local department store and purchase Velcro™ weights for your wrists and ankles. They can be found in 1 to 5 lb. (.5 to 2 kg) sizes. If you haven't exercised in a while, start with the 1 or 2 lb. (.5 or 1 kg) size and work your way up to 5 lb. (2 kg). Velcro weights increase the amount of fat you burn and help build nice, strong muscles effortlessly. That's what we all want—effortless muscle gain and fat loss. When I get up in the morning, I strap them on. I watch the news and lift my arms up and down throughout the program and, as a result, I have no more sagging skin on the backs of my arms—all while watching television. This is especially good for those of you who are not able to walk very far due to cardiovascular disease, diabetes, or arthritis.

Next, buy yourself a set of dumbbell weights. These are widely available. Usually they will have three different sizes. For women, start with the 3, 5, and 8 lb. (1.5, 2, and 3.5 kg) sizes. Men may need heavier weights. Don't start with weights that are too heavy or you may injure yourself or give up due to difficulty. To choose the correct weight for your ability, pick a weight that you think you can lift at least ten times without stopping. Pick up the dumbbell, bend your arm at the elbow, then lift the weight toward your shoulder. Do this ten times. If you can move the weight easily, you need a heavier weight. Add 2 or 3 lb. (1 or 1.5 kg). If you have a very hard time doing ten lifts, then you need a lighter weight. As you get stronger, you may have to add a couple of additional weights.

Rebounding for Stability and Cellulite Reduction

The rebounder, a small circular trampoline, is another inexpensive tool you can use to get fit. It usually stands about 8 inches (20.5 cm) off the floor and is about 36 inches (91.5 cm) around. It fits perfectly under your bed or in the back of your closet when not in use. I bought one for my kids when they were young (two years and up) so they could rebound in the playroom on rainy days. I have since reclaimed it. Ten minutes of rebounding is equivalent to thirty minutes of walking. And as long as you are not incontinent (leaking urine), it is a tremendous amount of fun. Some rebounders come with stability bars so you can hold on while you bounce—even those with poor balance can use it. The best thing about rebounding is that you will also exercise your lymphatic system, which drains and filters out dangerous substances and produces infection-fighting cells. The lymphatic system does not have a pump to perform cellular cleansing. You must exercise to promote movement through this system of vessels and tubes. One benefit of a healthy lymphatic system is cellulite reduction. Cellulite—skin like orange peel—forms when fluid distorts the cells in and around your fat and creates pockets in your skin. Women, because they have more fat, develop it more often than men. You will learn my fabulous cellulite-reducing tips in Chapter 8. Rebounding also creates muscle stability, essential to ensure that you do not fall or feel unstable as you age. Rebounding also benefits your cardiovascular system. Strap on your Velcro weights before you use the rebounder and get added weight-loss benefits. Rebounders are available at fitness stores and most department stores. Rebound during your favorite television show. No more guilt about watching television, because you are now multitasking.

Exercise Timing

One of the most common questions about working out is, "Should I work out in the morning or the evening?" The best time to perform the Body

Sense program is in the morning. Do ten minutes of this fun program and eat the recommended breakfast, and you will rev up your fat-burning furnace by 25–40 percent. The effects will last for twelve or more hours. You don't want to rev up your metabolism a few hours before you go to sleep. Plus, you want the added fat-burning action all day when we eat. Set your alarm ten minutes earlier and you will be rewarded with a tighter, stronger body. You know that all your good intentions of exercising after work will be dashed because you will be too tired to work out after making dinner and dealing with children. Consistency is the key. Get out of bed, put on a T-shirt and shorts, get your water bottle and towel, and get started. Exercise, then hit the shower, then eat breakfast. Start Day 1 on Monday so that Day 6 and Day 7 will be Saturday and Sunday, usually the days people don't go to work and do more outdoor or family-oriented aerobic activities.

Fitness Fun Ten Minutes a Day

Warm up before you begin. Stretch your arms to the ceiling. Breathe deeply. Then reach to the floor. Breathe deeply. Repeat 6 times. Jog in place for 30–60 seconds. Then lie on your belly and place your hands comfortably beneath your shoulders so you can push your chest off the floor and stretch your upper body toward the ceiling. This is not a push-up; it is more like a yoga position. You will be stretching your upper body muscles and elongating your back. Make sure to drink water so you are well hydrated before you begin, and remember to drink more water between the two sets of exercises. Dehydration can make you feel weak and dizzy.

The goal is to eventually do three sets of each exercise with successively heavier weights. Start with the lightest weight and work toward the heaviest. Depending on your level of fitness, you may be able to do this easily. Or you may be able to do only a few repetitions with the lightest weight. Whatever your level, you will build on your previous success, so if on Day 1 you can lift the weight only three times, then the next time try to do four repetitions. Then move on to a heavier weight, and so on, until you finally reach the goal of three sets of repetitions using successively heavier weights. The fact that you are trying is success. And remember, no matter what your age or fitness level, you will be able to do these exercises, so just have fun.

Body Sense Forty-Two-Day Program That Gives Results

For the next forty-two days you will do ten minutes of exercises each morning, five days a week, to achieve a stronger, sexier, fitter you. You will be surprised how quickly your body will respond by becoming more toned and shapely.

Week 1, Day 1

Shapely Arms

Stand with your feet shoulder-width apart. Hold a dumbbell in each hand. (Begin with the lightest weights.) Breathe in deeply, then exhale and curl both arms to a 90-degree angle. Make sure your elbows are at your sides and not bending outward. Hold for two seconds. Inhale as you lower the weights. If you are pushing your stomach out and bending backward, your weights are too heavy. Make sure you are standing straight and strong. Exhale and repeat ten times. Do not pause between curls. Next, pick up the medium weights and repeat ten curls. Then choose the heaviest weights and repeat ten curls. If you find that you cannot complete the last set of ten curls, then use the medium weights for both the second and third set of repetitions. It is best to do the required thirty curls even if you begin by using the smallest weights for all thirty. This exercise makes your neck muscles tighten up so your chin stops sagging.

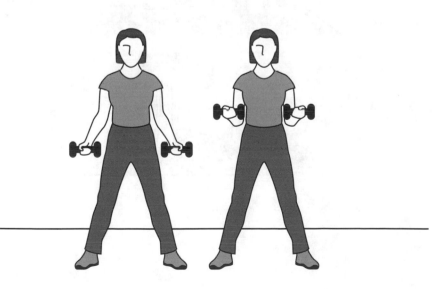

Arms without Wings

This exercise makes the backs of your arms beautiful while toning your abdominal muscles. Start with your lightest dumbbells. Lie on your back on the floor with your knees bent and the soles of your feet flat on the floor. Hold the dumbbells by your ears, with your elbows pointing up to the ceiling. Exhale as you raise the weight from your ears toward the ceiling. Push until your arms are straight up. Hold for two seconds and inhale as you lower the weights. Repeat ten times. Do not pause between curls. Next, choose the medium weights and repeat ten curls. Then use the heaviest weights and repeat ten curls. To really get the benefit of this exercise, hold your abdominal muscles tight and push your lower back toward the floor after you inhale. Focus on your breathing. If you can't complete all three sets with successively heavier weights, use the lightest dumbbells. Within a couple of weeks you will be able to progress to the heaviest weights.

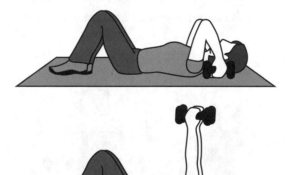

Week 1, Day 2

Sexy Calves

Stand tall with your feet shoulder-width apart. Hold the lightest dumbbells in your hands with your arms at your sides. Keep your shoulders back but relaxed. (Don't pull them up toward your ears.) Exhale as you raise your heels until you are on the balls of your feet. Keep raising your heels until you are on your tiptoes. Hold for two seconds. Inhale as you slowly lower your heels. Repeat for ten lifts. Next, pick your medium weights and repeat. Then use the heaviest weights and repeat for ten more lifts. Beautiful calves are the result of this exercise. Once the exercise becomes effortless, add Velcro weights to your ankles and continue to hold the dumbbells.

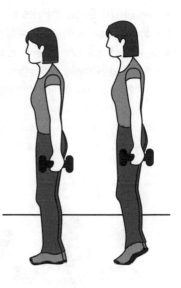

Tight Thighs and Cellulite Reducer

This exercise, called a squat, is my favorite: it gives the fastest results. Stand with your feet slightly wider than your shoulders, with your arms at your sides. Keep your back straight. Exhale as you squat down to about 90 degrees with your butt out as if you were going to sit down. Your knees should be in line with your toes. Hold for one or two seconds. Inhale as you straighten up. Do ten squats, then rest for a count of ten. Do ten more squats. Soon you will be able to do an additional ten squats for a full thirty squats. This exercise sculpts great legs and helps tighten the skin on your upper thighs and butt to reduce cellulite. Once you get very good at this exercise, add the Velcro™ weights to your wrists.

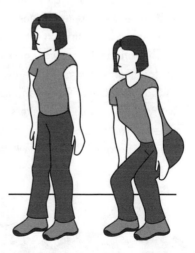

Week 1, Day 3

Chest and Breast Press

Lie on your back with your knees bent and the soles of your feet flat on the floor. Hold your lightest dumbbells with your arms out from your body like a cross. Bend your arms at the elbows, raising your hands toward the ceiling. Exhale as you push the weights toward the ceiling. Hold for a count of two and inhale as you bring the weights back to the starting position. Repeat for ten presses. Then change to your medium weights and repeat for ten presses. Finally, choose your heaviest weights and repeat. This exercise makes strong arms and builds chest muscles. It tightens sagging breasts in women.

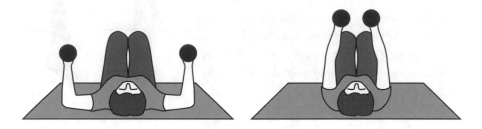

Tight Abdomen

You may be able to do only a few of these at the beginning, which is fine. Start slowly and add a few more repetitions every time you do the exercise. Always do as many as you can, up to ten in each set.

Lie on the floor on your back with your knees bent and the soles of your feet flat on the floor. Cross your arms over your chest. Exhale as you curl your upper body toward your knees. If you can raise your back only a few inches off the floor, don't worry—it will get easier. Make sure your lower back is not arched. Repeat as many times as you can. Remember, the more you do this exercise, the tighter your abdominals will become. The inches will fall off soon. You can do it.

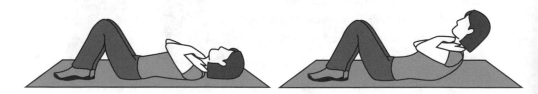

Week 1, Day 4

Butt Lift

Kneel on a rug or mat on all fours. You should have your hands and feet positioned so that you feel steady. While keeping your head up (do not look at the floor), exhale and raise your right leg until your thigh is level with your back and push your foot toward the ceiling. Hold for one second and inhale as you return your knee to the original position. Do ten repetitions for the right leg, then repeat for the left leg. This exercise gives you the greatest butt lift. When you can, increase the number of repetitions to fifteen per leg, then twenty.

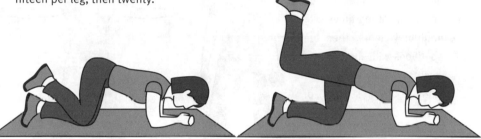

Even Better Butt Lift

Pick a sturdy chair and lie on the floor on your back with the chair at your feet. Place your palms flat on the floor with your arms at your sides. Lift your legs and put your heels firmly on the chair. Exhale as you contract the backs of your thighs and lift your butt toward the ceiling. Hold for two seconds. Inhale as you slowly lower your body back to the starting position. Do ten repetitions. Stop, rest for ten seconds, do ten more repetitions, rest, then do the last ten repetitions. Once you feel strong doing ten repetitions, add another five, and so on.

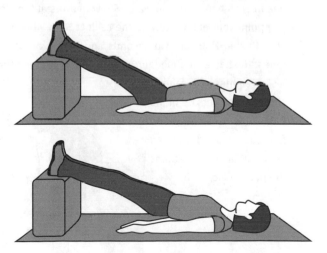

Week 1, Day 5

Shoulder Lift

Stand with your feet shoulder-width apart, your back straight, and your arms at your sides. Grip your lightest dumbbells one in each hand. With your palms facing the ceiling, raise your arms from your sides until they are level with your shoulders. When your arms are at shoulder height, turn your palms down and hold for one second. Inhale as you lower the weights. Repeat ten times. Repeat ten times with medium weights, then ten repetitions with the heaviest weights. If you feel yourself pushing out your stomach, or if you need to arch your back, your weights are too heavy. Use lighter weights or reduce the number of repetitions.

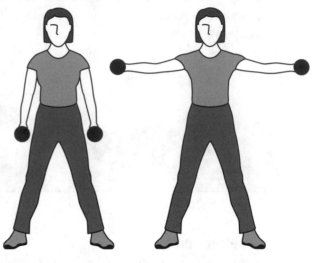

No More Back Fat

Sit in an armless chair. Put your lightest dumbbells on either side of the chair. Pick up one in each hand. Lean forward with your arms at the sides of the chair and exhale as you point your elbows toward the ceiling. Stop when your hands are at the height of your thighs. Hold for two seconds and inhale as you lower your arms. Repeat ten times. Next, use your medium weights and repeat ten times. Finally, choose the heaviest weights and repeat. This exercise gets rid of the flab women accumulate on the back around the bra strap; it also strengthens the back muscles.

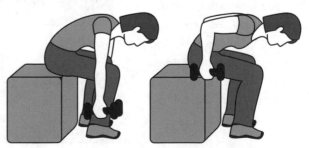

Week 1, Day 6 and Day 7

Go for a walk in the park, bicycle with your kids, swim, golf, play tennis, garden, or go dancing. Do anything that requires movement. You have done fabulous work and should be proud of yourself. Even after five days most people feel stronger and want to exercise. It is so easy to fit ten minutes of exercise into your day. If you miss a day because you slept through your alarm, just remember to do your exercises the next day. You will succeed with this program because it is easy.

Week 2, Day 1

Arms and Shoulders

Sit in an armless uncushioned straight-backed chair. Tighten your stomach muscles and keep your back straight. Hold one of your lightest weights in each hand. Raise your arms until they are even with your shoulders. Then bend your elbows to 90 degrees, pushing the weights toward the ceiling while exhaling. Hold for two seconds, then inhale as you lower the weights to shoulder height. Do ten repetitions if possible. This is a challenging exercise, so start with as many repetitions as you can do, building up to ten in a set. As you get stronger, do a second set of repetitions with your medium weights, then a third set with the heaviest weights. Your shoulders will get that lovely curve, your breasts will lift, and your arms will be strong.

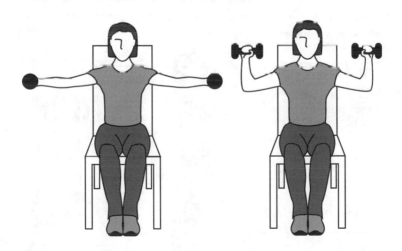

Shapely Arms

Stand with your feet comfortably apart. Hold a dumbbell in each hand, arms at your sides, elbows slightly bent forward. Lift the weight so your elbows bend into an L-shape. Hold for two seconds. Remember to exhale as you raise the weight and inhale as you return to the starting position. Do ten repetitions, then repeat with the medium weights. Do a final set with the heaviest weights.

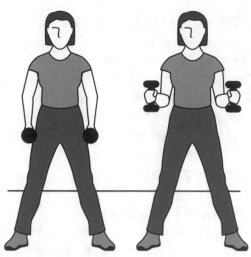

Week 2, Day 2

Slim Thighs

Stand straight with your hands at your sides. Step forward with your right leg and bend your knee in a 90-degree angle. Your knee should be above your foot. Hold this position for two seconds. Inhale as your return to the original position. You may be able to do only a few of these to begin with. That's fine. The key is to do this exercise with strength and precision; don't wobble. If you can do only two lunges with strength, then do two. Work up to ten repetitions for each leg. This exercise makes the tops of your thighs nice and shapely, and tightens your butt muscles and your abdominal muscles. You could eventually do the exercise holding your dumbbells or with Velcro weights.

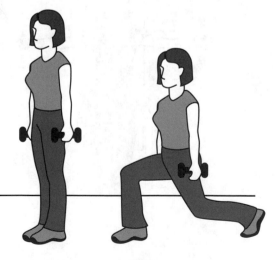

Inner Thigh

Lie on your side with your arm bent under you, supporting your upper body off the floor. Align your legs with your body. Inhale and then exhale and raise your leg toward the ceiling. Hold for two seconds. Initially you may not be able to lift it very high, but as you get stronger you will be able to lift your leg above your shoulder. Do ten repetitions. Repeat with the other leg. This exercise firms your thighs and stops them from rubbing together. Once you get good at this exercise, try it with your Velcro ankle weights.

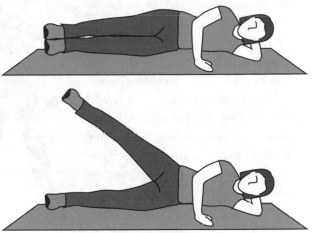

Week 2, Day 3

Back and Arms

Sit in an armless chair. Keep your back straight and hold one dumbbell in front of you with both hands. Your hold should be firm but comfortable. Exhale and lift the dumbbell over your head. Then inhale and move the dumbbell over the top of your head until your elbows are bent at a 90-degree angle and the dumbbell is behind your head. Hold for two seconds. Try to keep your elbows close to your head, but don't squeeze your head. Exhale then bring the dumbbell back over head. Repeat ten times. Move to the medium weight and repeat. Once you are strong, you will be able to complete three sets with a small, medium, and heavy weight. If you don't feel confident holding the weight above your head, do this exercise with your Velcro weights strapped on your wrists.

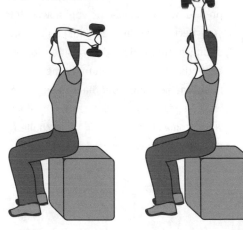

Shoulders, Arms, and Back

Stand with your back straight, your knees comfortably bent, and your feet about shoulder-width apart. Pick up a dumbbell in each hand, palms toward the floor. Let your arms hang straight down in front of your thighs. Bend your elbows slightly and raise the right dumbbell to eye level while exhaling. Inhale and slowly lower the dumbbell to your thigh. Repeat with the left arm. Do ten repetitions with each arm using the lightest weights. Then move to the medium weights and repeat ten times for each arm. Eventually you will be able to do another ten with the heaviest weights.

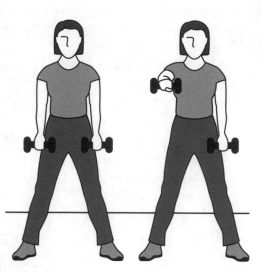

Week 2, Day 4

Great Legs

Stand with your back against the wall, your feet shoulder-width apart and your hands on your thighs. Exhale as you slowly slide your back down the wall until you are in a sitting position. Hold this position for two seconds. Inhale and return to the upright position, keeping your back against the wall. Repeat this exercise ten times. If you want to make this exercise more challenging, add Velcro weights to your wrists.

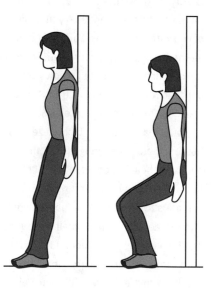

Better Butt

Stand with your feet apart in a comfortable position and your hands on your thighs. Squeeze your butt muscles and lower yourself into a sitting position. Hold for the count of two. Exhale and return to the upright position. Repeat this exercise ten times. Rest and repeat ten more times. Rest and repeat another ten times. You may be able to do only one set at first. As you get stronger, you will be able to complete the full three sets. When you get really good at this exercise, try it with Velcro weights on your wrists, or hold your dumbbells.

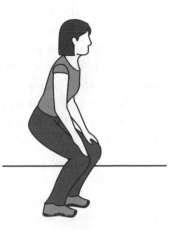

Week 2, Day 5

Long, Lean Leg Muscles

Stand beside a chair. Stand tall with your feet comfortably apart, your arms at your sides. Lift your right leg until your knee is bent at a 90-degree angle, then straighten your leg in front of you and hold it for two seconds. Do this exercise ten times, and then repeat with the other leg ten times. Repeat for a total of three sets for each leg. This exercise is designed to give you core balance. Once you become strong, add Velcro weights to your ankles and watch those leg muscles become lean and beautiful.

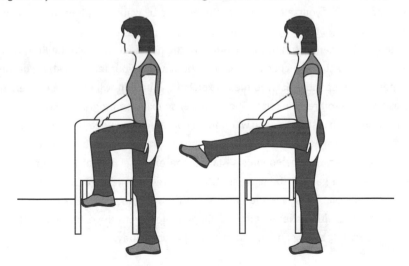

Flat Lower Abdominals

Kneel and place your hands firmly on the floor. Make sure your hips are above your knees and your shoulders are directly above your hands. Keep your back and tummy muscles in a relaxed position. Let your tummy sag down. Then gently use your stomach muscles to pull your belly button toward your lower spine. Hold for ten seconds. Then relax. Repeat this exercise ten times. This quickly fixes sagging lower abdominals.

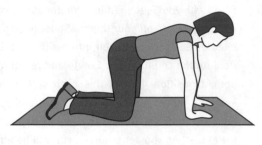

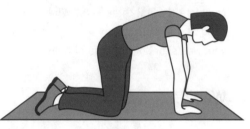

Week 2, Day 6 and Day 7

Have fun and spend time exercising with your family. You have just finished two weeks of amazing exercises, and I am sure by now your muscles are getting stronger. You should be proud of yourself. Accelerate the process by walking, riding your bike, gardening, and doing other physical activities.

Repeat the exercises in the same order for the next four weeks of the Body Sense program and watch the inches melt off your body while your muscles start showing. Your body will respond quickly to these exercises, your skin will become clearer, and you will be able to breathe better. The Body Sense exercise program is so easy to do and provides such fast results you will want to continue it every day for the rest of your life. People of all ages have been following this program for the past couple of years, and many women with osteoporosis started the exercise part of the program and made substantial gains in bone mass. Others have told me their cholesterol levels have dropped. Diabetics rave the most about this program, because the complications associated with diabetes start to disappear along with the extra weight. But the best part is feeling strong and fit and in control of your body.

EXERCISE AND KETOSIS

Most diets make you so weak you couldn't do even ten minutes of exercise per day. By the fourth day on the Body Sense diet, you will notice that you have more energy and stamina. Once you have eliminated the bad carbohydrates from your diet and have started eating the good carbohydrates along with healthy, fat-burning fats, proteins, and supplements, the cells that give you energy will start pumping, and your fat will start melting away. In the first two weeks of the Body Sense Natural Diet program, your body will start burning fat faster (a state called ketosis) and this, with exercise, provides fast weight loss.

Research as early as the 1980s showed that a diet made up of twenty-five percent carbohydrates not only significantly improved the rate at which people lost fat and lowered their cholesterol levels but also provided lots of energy. Research has also shown that a diet of only five percent carbohydrates increased strength and stamina and improved insulin levels. Bodybuilders and weightlifters have been using the ketosis/exercise technique for decades to get the best shape and maximum strength for competitions. All you want to do is get rid of that jiggling fat, and it is so simple using the Body Sense program. In forty-two days, you will agree.

Quick Strategies for Losing Weight, Gaining Muscles, and Reversing Disease

1. Put your favorite music in the CD player. Turn up the sound and start exercising. Sing while you exercise.
2. You are now exercising ten minutes every morning. Ideally, you are also doing some other activity such as walking, dancing, housecleaning, or gardening. Make sure you alternate higher-intensity workouts with lower-intensity workouts. For example, if you run 3 miles (5 km) on Monday, walk on Tuesday. Give your body time to recover and keep your immune system in balance.
3. Remember to take the stairs instead of the elevator, park your car far from the door of the office or shopping mall, and walk to the corner store instead of driving. Every little bit of exercise helps.
4. How hard you exercise during your workout is another component of success. Intensity, measured as a function of heart rate, ranges between

fifty-five and eighty-five percent of your maximum heart rate. Beginners will be around fifty-five percent; more active people will be closer to the upper limit. Whether you are a beginner or a serious athlete, one rule of thumb is that you should be able to talk while you are exercising. If you can talk easily as if nothing is going on, then you probably need to pump it up a little. If you are out of breath or wheezing, then slow down—you have pushed yourself too far too soon. If you get dizzy, stop exercising and visit your doctor to find out if your cardiovascular system is healthy.

5. If you are a beginner—for example, if you haven't exercised since your last high school physical education class—don't worry if you can't complete the ten-minute workouts. Do what you can. Even if all you can do is three minutes, just do it—and do it every day. Time yourself and add a minute every third workout. You will improve in the first few weeks.

6. Variety is the spice of life. To prevent boredom and injury, on your non-workout days, try different activities. Do something because it's fun, not just because it burns calories. Exercise should not feel like one more chore on your to-do list.

7. Follow the Body Sense food recommendations: take essential fatty acids (the fat-burning fats) and eat grapefruit, which contains naringin, a fat burner.

8. Eat breakfast every day. Get a good protein drink mix and add berries and yogurt to it. Eat PGX fiber-rich foods to fill you up.

9. Eat your meals on a smaller plate, or fill up your plate as you normally would and put half back.

10. Make sure you eat snacks as recommended in the Body Sense eating plan. Protein (one hard-boiled egg is loaded with pure protein) or low-carbohydrate snacks throughout the day will keep hunger pangs at bay.

11. Eat foods low on the glycemic index (see Chapter 2).

12. Take 5-HTP. It has been shown to curb appetite and increase serotonin, your feel-good hormone (see Chapter 6).

13. If you are tired and stressed, your cortisol levels will remain high throughout the day. High cortisol levels give you that spare tire around the middle. If you are exercising and eating correctly and you still can't budge the bulge, ask yourself if you are stressed and/or tired (see Chapter 4).

14. Take fat-burning nutrients (see Chapter 5). Drink lots of filtered water and herbal teas (see Appendix) Choose a tea rich in fat-burning catechins.
15. No white foods—no white bread, white pasta, white rice, white potatoes. No fake sugars like aspartame, and no non-dairy creamers. These foods are void of nutrition. They make you fat and increase the risk of diabetes.
16. Sleep. Take 3 mg of sublingual melatonin to aid restful, rejuvenating sleep.

Adopt as many of the recommendations as you can and watch your weight drop, your health improve, and your energy levels soar.

FITNESS TRAINERS

If you are one of those people who just can't seem to get motivated to exercise, or if you need someone to tell you what to do, fitness trainers are worth every penny they charge. They can develop a program with your health concerns in mind. Most important, they set a schedule and motivate you by meeting you at the gym. Their encouragement and support make working out more fun. Your local community center most likely has a fitness/workout room; many community centers have trained staff that can help you develop a safe program and show you how the equipment works. Many fitness clubs employ personal trainers. Check certification and ask for references.

Aerobic exercise without weight training will not burn fat, and weight training alone will not work, either. The key to fat burning is a combination of weight and cardiovascular training. The *American Journal of Cardiology* published a study comparing aerobic workouts to aerobic exercise with weight training. One group performed seventy-five minutes of aerobic exercise twice a week, while the second group did thirty-five minutes of weight training and forty minutes of aerobic exercise twice a week. Results were spectacular. The group that combined aerobics and weight training had as much as 43 percent more in overall strength and a 109 percent increase in endurance. The aerobics group had an 11 percent increase in endurance and no increase in strength. The reason: you need to build muscles to burn fat. Most of us don't enjoy huffing on the treadmill or the stair-climber for seventy-five minutes, anyway. Weight training is more fun and offers more variety. After two weeks of ten minutes per day of the Body Sense program, you will see amazing results on all the muscles worked.

EXERCISE AND IMMUNITY

You don't have to run on a treadmill for hours, and research is showing that excessive exercise (seen in exercise zealots, army recruits, and manual laborers) may be detrimental to your health and may speed up the aging process. To encourage your immune system to thrive, participate in moderate exercise as recommended in this book. Researchers in Toronto studied the effects of exercise on immunity in healthy young males. Each group was asked to do aggressive, aerobic activity for forty minutes per day. One group exercised five days of the week and the other group only three days per week. Blood tests revealed that the group exercising five days a week had lowered antibody production, thus showing weaker immune function. The group that exercised only three days a week demonstrated overall enhancement of their immune systems. Now this does not give you permission to reduce your activity, but it does show that everything in life is about balance.

Low to moderate exercise is beneficial to your health and enhances immunity. Walking is the most potent immune-enhancing activity: it provides movement and gives you a chance to clear your mind. Boost the intensity and duration of that same exercise by becoming a marathon runner, and you may find that too much of a good thing can be bad. If you exercise too much, you place stress on your immune system. You will catch more colds and flus, and it will take you longer to relax after exercising. Marathon runners and bodybuilders who work out without adequate rest or nutrients are especially prone to the negative effects of strenuous, relentless exercise.

Prominent immunologists and sports physiologists asked why marathon runners are prone to colds and influenza immediately after a marathon. Excessive physical stress causes tissue damage, which promotes an increase in the secretion of cortisol and pro-inflammatory factors.

Have you ever noticed that many marathon runners and other people who take part in excessively demanding, repetitive sports look aged? Without a good, solid diet and nutrient program, they are speeding up the aging process—muscles start to waste, and skin wrinkles and sags. The body will find the nutrients it needs, even if it has to steal them from muscles, bones, and connective tissues. Make sure you are getting enough nutrition for the energy you are expending.

SLEEP AND GET THIN

Sleep is essential to a healthy metabolism and helps prevent premature aging. If you are like most people, you go to bed too late, watch television in bed (which disrupts sleep), and wake up tired and groggy. During sleep your body regenerates. More important, if you do not sleep well every night, your hormones become disrupted. Research reported in the *Journal of the American Medical Association* in June 2002 found that even one week of mild sleep deprivation (characterized by the inability to fall asleep, frequent waking, or not enough hours of sleep) had a negative effect on hormone levels. In addition, results showed that a lack of sleep contributes to high blood pressure, heart disease, diabetes, and inflammation—all factors that will stop you from exercising and will ultimately lead to weight gain.

Tips for Sound Sleep

Sleep is essential to keeping your hormones balanced, allowing your body to regenerate, and providing you with the rest you need to energize for the next day. Sound, restful sleep is easy once you try some of the following tips:

- Do not take stimulants (coffee, pop, tea) after 3 p.m.
- Do not exercise after work. Exercise in the morning.
- Do not eat a big meal after 7 p.m.
- Take your calcium and magnesium supplement at bedtime.
- Take 3 mg sublingual melatonin at bedtime. Melatonin aids restful sleep, reduces your risk of certain cancers, resets your internal clock, and has a positive effect on growth hormone.
- Ensure that your room is free of light and your television is not left on while you sleep. Light inhibits melatonin production.
- Use the herbs valerian, chamomile, passion flower, or hops at bedtime to aid restful sleep.

- Avoid television or computer work, which stimulate the brain, at bedtime.
- Make a to-do list for tomorrow before you get to the bedroom so you will not run the list through your head while in bed.
- Take a hot bath at bedtime. Add 2 cups (500 mL) Epsom salts and 1 cup (250 mL) baking soda along with the essential oils of lavender or chamomile to detoxify and relax you.
- To calm the nerves, put a tissue moistened with lavender essential oil inside your pillowcase at bedtime.
- Relax. Breathe in through your nose and out through your mouth a few times while practicing the positive affirmations you learned in Chapter 3.

LIFE-GIVING WATER

After oxygen, water is the most essential nutrient. You could last months without food, but without water you would die in about a week. Your body is seventy-five percent water.

Dr. Fereydoon Batmanghelidj, author of *Your Body's Many Cries for Water*, says, "Most of us suffer from severe chronic dehydration, which is responsible for many of our illnesses. By drinking more water, we can cure ourselves of angina, rheumatoid arthritis, asthma, colitis, constipation, edema, gout, headaches (including migraines), hypertension, ulcers, obesity, fatigue, osteoporosis, and neck, muscle, and back pain." And your bouts of forgetfulness? Brain tissue is eighty-five to ninety percent water, and research documents that brain cells begin to shrink after prolonged dehydration. Water prevents aging. As you get older, your sense of thirst decreases, conspiring to prevent you from drinking what you need.

If you doubt the curative benefits of water, consider this: the body uses 7–11 qt (6.5–10.5 L) of water for the digestion of a meal, 3 pt (1.5 L) for saliva, 2 qt (2 L) for gastric juices, bile, and other secretions; the kidneys need 1 qt (1 L) of water for every 1.5 oz (45 mL) of waste removed; exhaling takes 1 pt (470 mL) each day, more if the climate is arid; and sweat uses up to 1 qt (1 L) of water an hour in dry conditions. Dr. Batmanghelidj's theory may not be so extreme.

You should drink at least six glasses of water daily. Thirst is a bad indicator; if you feel thirsty, you have already been dehydrated for far too long. Drink water even when you are not thirsty. Drink two glasses while performing your ten minutes of exercises, and keep large water bottles everywhere to remind you to take a sip—in the office, in the car, even on the table by your bed or favorite reading chair. Hot weather warrants doubling or tripling your intake. Remember, children need lots of water too. Encourage your whole family to drink water rather than juice (which contains too much fruit sugar) or artificial beverages such as pop, and instil this habit in your children while they are young. If you find plain water boring, add herbal tea bags to your water bottle. You could also add a little unsweetened cranberry or apple juice, or use lemon or lime to flavor the water—anything that will encourage you to drink more water. The only time you do not need to drink lots of water is while eating, as this dilutes your stomach acid and the digestive enzymes you need for digestion.

Water and Weight Loss

- Dehydration causes a decline in energy. You can't exercise if you have no energy.
- Dehydration makes you feel tired.
- Dehydration causes your blood volume to drop, making it harder for your heart to pump.
- Water makes you feel full.
- Water has zero calories.
- Water promotes movement of toxins out of and around cells, helping reduce cellulite.
- Water gives you energy.
- Water makes you alert.
- Water makes your skin beautiful.
- Water gets your bowels moving, helping to eliminate pounds of waste material.

CONCLUSION

Fitness has to be fun, or you won't do it. Ask yourself when you stopped exercising. Was it because you had a baby? Or did you stop when you started working overtime at your job? There is always a reason. Ask yourself why and then tell yourself you won't let anything get in your way of a flat stomach, better balance, and strong muscles.

Once you start the Body Sense program there will be no turning back. You will love seeing those rolls around your abdomen and the jiggling skin between your armpit and elbow disappear. You will start wearing short sleeves again and pants that don't have an elastic waistband. People will remark on how fabulous you look. They will want to know your secret. Ten minutes every morning along with great food—it is so easy to achieve with the Body Sense program.

Conquering Cellulite

Now that you are loosing weight and feel great you want it all   and that includes nice, smooth-looking skin. Rolls of fat and bulging, lumpy skin are often a side effect of the pounds you put on over the years. Now that Body Sense has created a thinner you, the excess fat is gone but lumpy, orange-peel-looking skin, known as cellulite, may still remain. If you have noticed lately that the skin on your buttocks, abdomen, thighs, neck, and upper arms is not as smooth as it used to be, you may have cellulite. According to the American Skincare and Cellulite Expert Association, approximately ninety percent of women older than twenty have cellulite and, contrary to popular belief, you do not have to be overweight to have cellulite, but if you are, the cellulite will be much worse. Diagnostic techniques, including ultrasonic liposculpturing and thermal imaging, have confirmed that cellulite is a medical condition, called lipodystrophy. A new field of medicine called aesthetic endocrinology has been evaluating the role of female hormones in the development of cellulite. Finally, cellulite is being taken seriously, as researchers and health care professionals understand it is associated with poor circulation and lymphatic drainage.

WHAT IS CELLULITE?

The word "cellulite" originates from the French word for cell with the suffix -ite, which means "disease." Thin women, overweight women, and normal-weight women can develop cellulite. You have most likely heard the term "orange-peel skin," used to describe how cellulite looks and feels. The appearance of lumps and bumps just below the skin's surface, has many women wearing long skirts or pants and covering their bottoms with towels when they're at the beach. Millions of dollars have been invested by the cosmetic industry to develop creams, lotions, and techniques to deal with this disfiguring condition. In the extreme cases, some work, but most don't. Some women are so devastated by the appearance of their skin that their self-esteem is damaged.

Women are more affected by cellulite because a woman's fat layer is organized differently than a man's. Most men store smaller amounts of fat deep under the skin, whereas women have an abundance of fat stored in the uppermost layer of the skin. Even thin women have fat. Fat is necessary to protect our bony protrusions from bumps and injury, to keep you insulated from cold, and to help you absorb vitamins A, D, and E.

Under your epidermis (skin) there are three layers of fat, and cellulite forms in the first layer, called the subcutaneous fat layer (hypodermis). Connective tissue holds the fat chambers in this area. Cellulite is mostly fat, but simply losing weight will not always eliminate the orange-peel appearance. Cellulite develops in steps. It starts with damage to your lymphatic drainage system caused by a poor diet and digestion, not enough protein in the diet, a lack of exercise or excessive activity, an accumulation of toxins, repeated weight loss and weight gain, hormone imbalance, aging, and/or a toxic liver.

CELLULITE CLASSIFICATION

Cellulite is classified into four categories by the Nurnberger-Muller Scale. Gently pinch a few inches of skin between your thumb and forefinger in the area of your buttocks, thighs, abdomen, or upper arms.

- *Stage Zero*: When you are standing naked in front of a mirror the skin does not appear dimpled, and there is no orange peel effect when you pinch the skin.
- *Stage One*: When you are standing naked in front of a mirror the skin does not appear dimpled, but when you pinch your skin, you have bumps and lumps.

- *Stage Two*: You can see dimpling or the orange peel appearance when you are standing naked in front of the mirror, but not when you lie down.
- *Stage Three*: You can see dimpling on the skin when you are standing and lying down.

HOW CELLULITE DEVELOPS

Cellulite is formed when the drainage system in your fat cells becomes damaged. The drainage system fails to remove excess fluid, which accumulates in and around the connective tissue that holds the fat cells in place. Free radicals created by the stagnant flow of lymph cause damage to surrounding capillaries, veins, and connective tissue. Blood flow, oxygen, and nutrition to cells in the surrounding area are reduced. Fat cells are pulled in different directions and they cluster together, distorting collagen (the "glue" that supports skin, tendons, bone, cartilage, and connective tissue) and connective tissue; fat and fiber accumulate where they should not. Normal cell function would not allow this to happen, but disordered pathways for lymph circulation allow a buildup of fibers and free radicals causing damage to the support systems of the skin to occur.

Areas of the body that accumulate cellulite—including the thighs, hips, abdomen, buttocks, upper arms, and the back of the neck—also have a higher number of fat cells. Once cellulite forms, your fat cells become distorted and may not release fat properly. They store more fat, becoming larger and larger, furthering the problem of poor lymph drainage and extensive fibrous tissue formation.

If cellulite is not dealt with, the affected skin may become so damaged it feels cold to the touch, alternating with hot zones where blood circulation is highly concentrated. When cellulite is fully entrenched, some people develop large fatty lumps under the skin, particularly on the front of the thighs just above the knees.

"Football player's legs," also called "footballer's legs" or dysmorphism, is an extreme cellulite condition affecting the fronts of the thighs. It is seen mainly in men and athletes of both sexes who exercise their legs excessively without working other areas of the body. Excessive use of the stair-climber, bike riding, running, or leg weight exercises can worsen this type of cellulite. I have seen this in women who had a problem with cellulite in their thighs and decided to do leg-based exercise in hopes of eliminating the problem, only to find that excessively exercising one spot makes it far worse. Everything is always about balance—no one type of exercise will eliminate cellulite. Cellulite is caused by the following:

- A diet devoid of vegetables
- Fat gain
- Yo-yo dieting (repeated weight loss and gain)
- High sugar consumption
- Liver congestion caused by toxin overload
- Inadequate consumption of protein, which causes water retention
- Lack of vitamins and minerals
- Poor digestion
- Poor insulin regulation in the body due to high-carbohydrate diet
- Lack of exercise
- Excessive repetitive exercise of the legs without exercising other areas
- Excessive caffeine and alcohol consumption
- Smoking, which impairs circulation
- Stress, which leads to high cortisol levels
- Pregnancy (because of its increased pressure on the lymphatic and venous systems and because of weight gain)
- Adrenal exhaustion, causing a craving for salt, which promotes excess water retention
- Untreated food allergies
- Consumption of artificial sweeteners
- Estrogen imbalance, especially during menopause or perimenopause
- Hysterectomy, which could impair lymph flow
- Constipation, hemorrhoids, and varicose veins, which put pressure on the lymph system
- Repeated air travel, which impedes the flow of lymph and blood

ESTROGEN AND CELLULITE

Estrogen has a direct effect on the metabolism of skin and hair, changes in body composition, and alterations of subcutaneous fat distribution throughout your life. Aesthetic endocrinology is a new field that looks at how an excess or a deficiency of estrogen contributes to obesity and cellulite.

Excess estrogen (also called estrogen dominance) creates a host of health problems in women, including endometriosis, uterine fibroids, fibrocystic breasts, breast cancer, ovarian cysts, heavy periods, estrogen belly, low thyroid, and fat deposits. Excess estrogen is thought to be the culprit that causes cellulite to build up around the fat cells and restrict lymphatic drainage and blood flow.

At menopause, the decline in estrogen promotes cellulite. It seems that too much or too little estrogen can create problems with connective tissue and can cause skin aging, lack of elasticity in the skin, and sagging skin. An excess of estrogen in the younger years, followed by a rapid decline at menopause, can cause cellulite to become extreme in the years after menopause.

Estrogen Mimickers

Environmental estrogens, also called "estrogen mimickers" and "xeno-estrogens" (pronounced "zeno estrogens"), further exacerbate the estrogen overload. These toxic estrogens are found in common everyday substances—plastics, pesticide-laden foods, deodorants, nail polish, cosmetics, foods containing dioxins (meat, milk, eggs, and fish), glues and adhesives—and they disrupt your estrogen balance, which leads to weight gain, poor thyroid function, and cellulite.

Fortunately, keeping your estrogens healthy and balanced is possible even when you are exposed to a daily onslaught of environmental estro gens. Eat only organic foods, because pesticide-laden fruits and vegetables are the main source of xenoestrogens. Choose cruciferous veggies—Brussels sprouts, broccoli, cauliflower, and kale—which contain plant nutrients that help keep your estrogens healthy and your hormones balanced. If you eat animal products, drink organic milk and eat organic yogurt, cheese, and beef; cows on non-organic farms are fed grains that have been sprayed with pesticides (xenoestrogens), and those pesticides become concentrated in their milk and meat. Don't use bleached feminine hygiene pads and tampons; the bleaching chemicals act as estrogen mimickers. Go to the health food store and buy unbleached feminine hygiene products. Do not microwave foods in plastic; use only glass or ceramic containers. Estrogen mimickers lurk in plastics; when those plastics are heated they release toxins. Take the following six nutrients to help keep

estrogen healthy, balance your hormones, detoxify, and eliminate carcino-
genic estrogens:

- Indole-3-carbinol
- Calcium D-glucarate
- Green tea extract
- Curcumin (turmeric)
- Milk thistle
- Sulforaphane

Indole-3-Carbinol

Indole-3-carbinol (I3C) is a plant nutrient found in broccoli, Brussels
sprouts, cauliflower, kale, and cabbage. Research has shown that I3C helps
break down cancer-causing estrogens into non-toxic forms and eliminates
harmful estrogen mimickers. I3C improves detoxification of the cyto-
chrome P450 enzyme system, which helps remove excess estrogen and/or
xenoestrogens. I3C has other benefits:

- I3C improves the ratio of good estrogens to toxic cancer-causing forms of
  estrogen.
- I3C protects against estrogen-dominant cancers, for example, breast and
  ovarian cancer.
- I3C reduces tumor development in the endometrium and cervix
- I3C inhibits the growth of prostate cancer cells.
- I3C and Tamoxifen™, (a drug used to block estrogen) work together to
  inhibit the growth of estrogen-dominant cancers more effectively than
  Tamoxifen abre.
- The human papilloma virus, which can lead to cervical cancer, uses a
  toxic form of estrogen (16-alpha-hydroxyestrone) to develop into cancer.
  Research has shown that abnormal Pap tests can be improved when
  women take I3C. In one study, thirty women with CIN II and CIN III cervical lesions called cervical intraepithelial neoplasia (CIN) took 200 mg
  or 400 mg of I3C daily. Fifty percent of women in the treatment group
  had complete regression of their lesions and normal Pap smears. None
  of the placebo group had any changes.
- Indole-3-carbinol balances healthy estrogens in the body and supports
  liver hormone function. Remember, your fat cells manufacture estrogen,

and excess estrogen contributes to weight gain. By using I3C, you can maintain proper estrogen function in your fat cells.

Recommended dosage: 150–300 mg per day.

Calcium D-Glucarate

Calcium D-glucarate is found in all fruits and vegetables; the highest concentrations are in apples, grapefruit, and broccoli. Calcium D-glucarate is a powerful detoxifier and removes excess estrogens from the liver, which is important for weight loss, liver health, and cellulite reduction. It metabolizes fats and keeps estrogen levels balanced. Its other benefits include:

- Calcium D-glucarate has been shown to reduce total triglyceride levels by an average of twelve percent, reducing the risk of cardiovascular disease and helping the body metabolize fats.
- It removes excess estrogens and xenoestrogens.
- It supports the liver.
- It inhibits tumor formation caused by chemical cancer-causing agents.
- In animal studies, calcium D-glucarate resulted in a fifty to seventy percent reduction of breast tumor formation.

Recommended dosage: 150–300 mg per day.

Green Tea Extract

Green tea extract is a powerful antioxidant containing polyphenols, catechins, and flavonoids, which have been shown to protect against estrogen-dominant conditions and related cancers, especially breast, ovarian, and prostate cancers. Green tea extract has been extensively studied for its weight-loss benefits. It keeps estrogen balanced. Its benefits include:

- Green tea extract increases the activity of other antioxidants.
- It inhibits cancer by blocking the formation of cancer-causing compounds.
- It increases detoxification of cancer-causing agents.
- It prevents breast and prostate cancers.
- It is essential for weight loss and cellulite reduction.

Recommended dosage: 100–200 mg per day. Buy green tea extract that has at least sixty percent polyphenols, an important active ingredient. Drink green tea throughout the day instead of coffee for maximum cellulite reduction.

Curcumin (Turmeric)

Curcumin is the yellow pigment of turmeric, one of the chief ingredients in curry. It is a powerful anti-inflammatory agent and inhibits all steps of cancer formation: initiation, promotion, and progression. Curcumin also helps eliminate cancer-causing estrogens and environmental estrogens via the liver. Curcumin increases detoxification. Its other benefits include:

- It is a potent antioxidant that squelches free-radical production in people with cellulite.
- It enhances glutathione, the most powerful detoxifier of the liver.
- It detoxifies the liver of cancer-causing substances, including environmental estrogens (pesticides and herbicides).
- It directly inhibits tumor growth.
- It deactivates cancer-causing agents.

Recommended dosage: 50–100 mg per day. Ensure that your curcumin supplement contains ninety-five percent curcumin. Use the spice turmeric in cooking, too.

Milk Thistle

Milk thistle, called the protector of the liver, is extremely important for cellulite reduction and proper estrogen balance in the body's cells. Its active ingredients include silybin, silydianin, and silychristin, collectively known as silymarin. Milk thistle enhances detoxification of toxic estrogen from the liver. It also has other powerful benefits, including:

- It detoxifies a wide range of hormones, drugs, and toxins.
- Milk thistle improves estrogen balance by metabolizing estrogen to the good estrogens.
- It stimulates growth of new liver cells.
- A powerful antioxidant and free-radical scavenger, milk thistle is several times more potent than vitamins E and C.

- It promotes bile flow for healthy digestion and gut health.
- It increases intracellular glutathione (necessary for detoxification) by thirty-five percent in healthy people.
- It has been researched for use in psoriasis, suppressed immune function, gallbladder disease, hepatitis, atherosclerosis, and alcoholic liver disease.
- It is necessary for cellulite reduction.
- It reduces the toxic effects of chemotherapy.
- It directly inhibits breast cancer cell growth.

Recommended dosage: 50–100 mg per day. Ensure that your milk thistle supplement contains at least eighty percent silymarin.

Sulforaphane

Sulforaphane, from broccoli sprout extract, has been shown to stimulate the body's production of detoxification enzymes that eliminate toxic estrogens. It also balances estrogens in the body. It is a powerful antioxidant and fights cancer. Its benefits include:

- Sulforaphane helps liver detoxification, important for detoxifying excess estrogens and environmental estrogens.
- Sulforaphane neutralizes dangerous carcinogens before they can damage DNA and promote cancer.

Recommended dosage: 200–400 mcg per day.

For All Women

Who needs these hormone-balancing and environmental estrogen-detoxifying nutrients? All women need these nutrients, especially those with cellulite. These nutrients are also especially important for women with the following conditions or those who want to prevent these conditions:

- estrogen-dominant conditions, including endometriosis, uterine fibroids, breast cancer or ovarian cancer
- ovarian cysts
- polycystic ovarian disease
- premenstrual syndrome

- perimenopause, excessively heavy periods, and unbalanced hormones
- excess weight (more harmful environmental estrogens are stored in fat)
- cellulite
- high cholesterol
- fibrocystic breast disease

CELLULITE-BUSTING TIPS

If you are overweight, losing weight is important, but don't be discouraged if your cellulite is still visible after you have lost 10 lb. (4.5 kg). The fat accumulations within the cellulite are usually the last fat to be eliminated. The following cellulite-busting strategies will ensure that you get rid of the cellulite you have and prevent it from returning.

What You Eat

The Body Sense Natural Diet program you have been following is perfect for reducing cellulite. Good, clean sources of protein, plenty of low-glycemic index vegetables, and essential fatty acids will help remove all of these stubborn deposits. A diet deficient in protein causes water retention, reduced cellular repair, and cellulite.

Eliminating all caffeine will speed up your cellulite-reducing program. Caffeine used topically on the skin has been found to enhance the elimination of cellulite, but too much caffeine taken internally constricts blood vessels and promotes cellulite.

Cellulite-Cleansing Juice

1	large head of Romaine lettuce	1
1/4	English cucumber with skin removed	1/4
1	small piece of ginger	1
1	small carrot	1
3	large celery stalks	3
	fennel, parsley, or favorite vegetable to taste	

Use organic vegetables wherever possible. Put all ingredients through the juicer and drink immediately. This is a refreshing juice and enhances detoxification.

Unsweetened pomegranate, cranberry, and blueberry juice can be purchased at the health food store and some grocery stores. These are excellent detoxification juices and I recommend that you mix them half and half with sparkling mineral water, add a twist of lime, and use them as a substitute for the fruit in one of your protein shakes as recommended in the Body Sense Natural Diet.

DETOXIFICATION BATHS

Detoxification baths use hot water to increase blood flow to the skin's surface and open the pores, thereby encouraging perspiration and toxin elimination. Start the baths slowly, take only one a week, then two, and so on, as you may experience symptoms, especially if your toxic load is great. If you experience dizziness, headaches, fatigue, nausea, or weakness during a bath, get out of the tub. Next time, bathe for a shorter period in cooler water. To take a detoxification bath: Fill the tub with water as hot as you can tolerate. (Filtered water is best. Filters for your showerhead are inexpensive and available at some health food stores and hardware stores.) Begin with a five-minute soak. Gradually increase your time in the detoxification bath to thirty minutes if you are not experiencing any symptoms. After soaking, shower and wash thoroughly with soap to rinse off toxins that have accumulated on the skin. Drink at least two or three glasses of purified water before, during, and after your bath.

Epsom Salts Baths

Epsom salts baths help eliminate toxins by increasing the blood supply to the skin and by drawing toxins from the body. Epsom salts contain sulfur, which is well known for its medicinal and detoxification properties. Add 1 cup (250 mL) Epsom salts to a regular bath and gradually increase the amount to 4 cups (1 L) per tub. Stay in an Epsom salts bath no longer than half an hour. Other substances you can add to the Epsom salts bath to help detoxification include:

- Apple cider vinegar, which works similarly to Epsom salts. Add 1 cup (250 mL) to your bath, gradually increasing to 2 cups (500 mL) per tub.
- Baking soda (sodium bicarbonate) added to a bath used to be a common household remedy for colds, flus, and skin irritations. Baking soda is good for cleansing the body. Use 1 cup (250 mL) baking soda per tub.
- Green clay, available at day spas and health food stores. Clay draws out toxins through the skin. Use 1/2 to 1 cup (125 to 250 mL) clay per tub.
- After your bath, dilute oil in a small amount of carrier oil, for example,

almond. Good essential oils to choose are peppermint, eucalyptus, cajeput, wintergreen, juniper, and clove. Apply to your skin after your bath. Gently massage the oil into the area affected by cellulite. These oils increase circulation and blood flow to the area.

SAUNAS AND STEAM MELT CELLULITE

Sweating is good for you! The primary storage site for toxins is fatty tissue. The heat generated during exercise removes toxins from the fat, while the increase in blood flow moves them into general circulation. The same holds true for saunas and steam baths. Heavy perspiration from exercise and saunas aids elimination of toxins from your body. Studies that measured chemical and heavy-metal levels in the sweat and blood during and after a sauna or exercise confirm the effectiveness of these methods for removing toxic chemicals from the body. The research indicates that sweating confers the following benefits:

- High body temperatures (fevers) combat the growth of viruses or bacteria and strengthen the immune system. Saunas have similar effects.
- Sweating burns calories and speeds up the metabolic processes of the detoxification and hormonal systems.
- Sweating speeds the breakdown of cellulite by aiding the movement of toxins, wastes, and blocked fat.
- Sweating excretes toxins and metabolic wastes from the body, including cadmium, lead, nickel, sodium, and excess cholesterol.
- Sweating in a hot environment such as a sauna will successfully remove chemical pollutants—PCBs, excess estrogens, and dioxins—that accumulate in fat cells.
- Sweating stimulates dilation of the blood vessels that lie close to the skin. This dilation relieves pain and speeds the healing of sprains, strains, bursitis, and arthritis, to name a few.
- Sweating promotes relaxation. In athletes, it improves recovery time after intense training sessions.

A detoxification sauna should be preceded by twenty minutes of exercise and followed by a cleansing shower. You can lose up to 4 cups (1 L) of water during a twenty-minute sauna, so be sure to replace lost fluids. Do not spend more than thirty minutes in a sauna.

There are two types of saunas: dry and wet. Dry saunas are preferred for detoxification because they increase the rate of natural sweating, speeding up the detoxification process more than the water-saturated air of a steam room can. You sweat more and faster in a dry sauna.

Dry Brushing

Dry brushing the skin prior to a sauna, detoxification bath, or shower removes dead skin and improves circulation to the skin, helping open the pores for elimination of toxins and cellulite. Use a skin brush made of soft, natural, nonabrasive bristles, available at most health food or beauty product supply stores. Do up to five minutes of long strokes over every area of your body, always moving toward your heart. For example, start at your feet and brush toward your heart. Then start with your buttocks, stomach, and chest and brush toward your heart.

CASTOR OIL PACKS

Castor oil from the castor bean plant *Ricinus communis* has been used therapeutically since ancient times; pharmaceutical and medical references to castor oil date back to the seventeenth century. Castor oil is used topically in a castor oil pack to enhance the functioning of the lymphatic system and the immune system. It is also a powerful detoxifier, drawing toxins out of the body from as deep as 4 inches (10 cm) below the surface. (This means they can be used to break up cellulite.) To make a castor oil pack, you will need:

- a large wool or flannel cloth (I use an old flannel sheet, cut up)
- plastic wrap
- a bath towel
- pure, cold-pressed free castor oil
- a hot water bottle
- old clothes

To make the pack, fold the flannel cloth so it is six layers thick. Pour enough castor oil onto the cloth so the cloth is wet but not dripping. Lie on an old sheet or towel and apply the cloth to the area you wish to detoxify, then cover the pack with the plastic wrap. Apply gentle heat from the hot water bottle for at least one hour.

If you want to sleep while using the pack, apply the pack, cover with plastic, wrap a towel around the entire area, and secure it with ties or pins. The pack should be applied for a minimum of one hour. For general detoxification, apply the pack over the liver area, from below the right nipple straight down to the waist. Wipe the skin after treatment. Castor packs can be applied daily. You may keep the cloth pack in a plastic container for future use, adding more castor oil as the cloth dries out. Castor oil pack treatments are essential in helping break up cellulite.

LYMPHATIC DRAINAGE

Your lymphatic system circulates lymph fluid throughout your body. That fluid carries toxic wastes and bacteria to lymph nodes, where the toxins are engulfed and destroyed by cells of the immune system. It is especially important for detoxification, cellulite treatment, and prevention of disease that the lymphatic system remains decongested. Lymphatic massage can be done daily to help facilitate detoxification.

EFFECTIVE EXERCISES TO REDUCE CELLULITE

Ten minutes of weight-bearing exercise each morning will improve skin tone, get your lymphatic system moving, and break down the irregular connective tissue and fat found in cellulite. Do not try to spot-reduce cellulite by overexercising one area. Variety is the key—weight-bearing exercises, walking, dancing, gardening, and swimming, all provide benefits to reducing cellulite. Rebounding is another effective method of dislodging cellulite (see Chapter 7). You cannot eliminate cellulite without exercise. Remember that even very thin women can develop cellulite. Exercise revives a sluggish lymphatic system and improves circulation to remove cellulite.

Massage Instructions for Lymphatic System

Most of the lymph vessels are located alongside veins and flow toward the heart. The main lymphatic duct empties into a vein near the top of the chest. Tightness or imbalance in the action of the upper chest muscles causes decreased chest expansion, thus putting pressure on this duct and decreasing the lymph flow. By massaging the areas in the order indicated by the numbers in the figure, you will stimulate and stretch these muscles, increase your rib cage expansion, and allow freer flow of lymph. You may find that your chest is tender at first, but the tenderness will diminish with consistent treatment, indicating that lymph flow is improving.

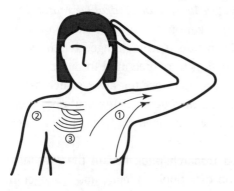

1. Lift one arm over the head, as shown. With the opposite hand, massage upwards from mid-chest to shoulder and along the side of the chest in the direction of the arrows, using the heel of your hand. Alternate strokes on both sides of the breast for twenty strokes. Then repeat the massage on the other side of the body.
(Note: Some people find this easier to do if the back is supported. If that is the case, stand against a wall, sit in a chair with good back support, or lie on a bed while doing the massage.)
2. Use the thumb or fingers to rub back and forth deeply and briskly under the tip of the shoulder.
3. Find the tops of the first three ribs, just below the collarbone. Rub along the tops of these ribs from the center of the chest to the outer edge of the chest for at least one minute on each side.
4. Massage all areas twice daily for one week, then once per day for a second week. After that, treat yourself to a massage every time you shower.

(*Source*: Reprinted with permission from Karen Jensen, N.D., and Lorna R. Vanderhaeghe, *No More HRT: Menopause, Treat the Cause*, 2002.)

TOPICAL TREATMENTS
Cellulite is a complicated condition, and cosmetic companies that advertise a quick-fix product are most likely exaggerating. An anticellulite cream alone will not break down these stubborn deposits, but good food, exercise, and

detoxification, combined with a good-quality topical cellulite product that promotes blood flow and metabolizes fats, will speed up the process. Clinical studies are proving the many benefits of these topical creams.

Research published in the *American Journal of Clinical Dermatology* in November 2000 found that topical application of retinol, a vitamin A acid, improved the appearance of the skin in fifteen women, aged twenty-six to forty-four, who had requested liposuction to reduce mild to moderate cellulite. Liposuction is an invasive surgery and does not always successfully deal with cellulite, which is a sign of a disordered detoxification system. The six-month study found that retinol improved the skin, promoting a smooth outer surface.

Double-blind, placebo controlled research published in the *Journal of Cosmetic Science* using a combination of retinol, caffeine, and ruscogenine (commonly known as butcher's broom) found that the topical application of these products reduced the orange-peel effect and increased circulation deep in the skin layers. The combination was found to be superior to placebo (fake pill).

Gota Kola

Gota kola (*Centella asiatica*) is used to treat weak veins (blood pools in the legs, causing aching pain, heaviness, swelling, and unsightly veins). Varicose veins and hemorrhoids are also treated using gota kola. It works by strengthening connective tissue and the walls of veins and capillaries, thus preventing and treating cellulite and other skin conditions such as keloid scars. By strengthening tissues, it inhibits leakage of fluid into surrounding tissues, which is how cellulite begins. Gota kola helps keep the thick fibrous cellulite tissue from forming around fat cells. It is excellent for advanced and profuse cellulite. Most good cellulite creams contain this herb.

Caffeine

Applied topically, caffeine is readily absorbed into the skin. It stimulates the fat cells to release fat. Several research studies have shown that the topical application of caffeine effectively metabolizes fat in those with cellulite.

Retinol

Retinol is a vitamin A acid used to treat fine wrinkles, acne, and, recently, cellulite. Retinol increases the rate at which the skin cells are renewed and helps the skin function properly. One study found that the combination of retinol and caffeine, used topically on areas affected by cellulite, produced a visible reduction in orange-peel skin. Participants in the study lost an average of nearly 1 inch (2.5 cm) around their waists.

Butcher's Broom

Butcher's broom is used to flush excess water from the body. It is also used topically and orally to treat hemorrhoids, weak veins, varicose veins, and cellulite. The plant contains anti-inflammatory substances that cause the contraction of blood vessels, especially veins. Use of this herb is not recommended for people with high blood pressure.

SPECIFIC CELLULITE SUPPLEMENTS

Many supplements are tailored to beat cellulite. Let's look at a few.

L-carnitine

L-carnitine, a potent fat-dissolving substance, is a vitamin-like nutrient with a structure similar to an amino acid (which is part of protein). There are more than 10,000 academic research papers on this amazing nutrient. While it burns up fat deposits, it helps detoxify and optimize cell metabolism. L-carnitine helps maintain healthy blood sugar levels, essential to effective weight loss.

Its cellulite-busting action occurs because it promotes circulation in the legs, aids the breakdown of waste products, and improves the fluidity of the blood, thus reducing deposits in veins and capillaries while enhancing metabolism. You need approximately 1–5 g of L-carnitine per day to break up cellulite and aid weight loss. It comes in capsule, tablet, and drink form.

Silicon

Silicon is an essential element required for the normal growth, development, and integrity of healthy bones, joints, hair, nails, and connective tissue. Every part of the body that requires strength and elasticity requires silicon.

Inadequate silicon intake has been associated with weak, brittle nails, weakened capillaries and arteries, and cellulite. This is because the protein matrix surrounding these areas is deficient in silicon. Look for silicon that is biologically active, as this is the only form of the essential element that is absorbed directly through the stomach wall and the gastrointestinal tract into the bloodstream (see Appendix A). Clinical studies confirm that biologically active silicon offers superior absorption and increases collagen concentration in the skin.

Slimming Tea

Use slimming teas with the following ingredients:

• *Garcinia Cambogia Extract*: Garcinia extract comes from India and has been extensively researched and used as one of the most successful weight-management herbs since the early 1970s. The active ingredient, hydroxycitric acid (HCA), has been shown to reduce the amount of lipids stored in the fat cells or as cholesterol. Garcinia converts much of this material into usable energy, creating a mild thermogenic action (heat) while increasing metabolic rate. When you increase heat and metabolic rate, you can burn off fat more effectively.

• *Hibiscus Flowers*: Hibiscus flowers are used as a gentle diuretic and for disorders of circulation. This herb is also useful as a treatment for constipation; it produces a very mild laxative effect.

• *Chinese Green Tea*: Green tea's mild stimulating action is well known for emulsifying lipids and enhancing digestion. Traditional Chinese medicine says that food stagnation plays a central role in weight gain. If you assist food digestion and absorption, you will desire less food, and excesses will be eliminated from your digestive tract. For centuries, Asians have used the combination of green tea and hawthorn berries to reduce excess fat.

• *Hawthorn Berry*: Hawthorn berries are used to reduce excess fat, strengthen the heart, and reduce blood lipids. The herb has a mild diuretic action.

• *Malva Verticillata Leaves*: This herb provides a soothing diuretic effect and promotes optimal performance of the digestive tract.

• *Parsley Root*: Parsley root is an effective diuretic and also promotes digestion.

• *Lemon Peel*: A slimming agent, lemon peel helps the body cleanse by promoting perspiration and acting as a natural diuretic. Lemons also aid digestion and reduce hyperacidity in the stomach.

• *Citric Acid*: Citric acid, extracted from citrus fruits, promotes movement of waste through the intestinal tract and adds flavor to tea.

• *Cranberries*: Well known as an effective preventive against and treatment for bladder infections, cranberries are a source of tannins. Cranberries are a gentle diuretic, helping to mobilize excess water retained in cells, a condition commonly found in people with cellulite.

CONCLUSION

Now that you are taking detoxification baths and/or saunas, have completed the 7 day detoxification diet and learned so much about your liver, digestion, nutrition and exercise, you will see those stubborn cellulite deposits melt away. After as little as 7 days you will also notice that the skin on your face and neck are glowing with health too. Now go shopping and buy those short sleeved shirts and leg-bearing shorts and skirts. Throw away the wrap you used to cover up your legs when wearing a bathing suit because your skin is gorgeous. You should be so proud of yourself for applying all the aspects of the Body Sense natural diet program and reaching your goals of a fitter, slimmer, healthier you.

Natural Treatment for Diabetes

We have covered a lot of ground in this book and now you know how important your food and lifestyle choices are to your overall health and weight management. It is my hope that what you have learned will change the way you live and feel permanently. I would be remiss, however, if I did not provide prevention and treatment strategies for diabetes in this book. You may be struggling with diabetes or have a friend or family member who is living with this dangerous and potentially deadly disease. There are two main types of diabetes. I will focus on preventing and treating Type 2 diabetes; being overweight is the number one risk factor for developing this form of diabetes. The recommendations in this chapter are designed to help you prevent and reverse Type 2 diabetes naturally.

According to the American Diabetes Association, fifty to ninety percent of people with Type 2 diabetes are overweight. Being overweight causes some degree of insulin resistance, the first step in developing Type 2 diabetes. The bottom line is that excess body fat causes Type 2 diabetes. Type 2 diabetes is a disease that is the result of an unhealthy diet and lifestyle. Nutritional strategies and exercise have been shown to reduce the risk of developing diabetes by fifty-eight percent. In some diabetics, the use of insulin and other diabetes medications was reduced or eliminated when nutritional treatment was added. If nothing else, the side effects associated with diabetes—including blindness, neuropathy, high cholesterol, heart disease, kidney disease, impotence, loss of circulation, and amputations—can be reduced or avoided using natural medicines alone or in combination with diabetes drugs.

In 2002 the World Health Organization estimated that more than 177 million people worldwide have diabetes. By 2025, this figure will top 300 million. More than 2 million Canadians have diabetes. In the United States, 18.2 million people, or 8 percent of the population, have diabetes. Of those with diabetes, it is estimated that up to 80 percent will die as a result of heart disease or stroke. It is also estimated that another 2 percent of people have diabetes and do not know it.

Diabetics secrete little or no insulin; and/or their bodies do not respond appropriately to insulin. This means they cannot transfer glucose from the bloodstream into cells and maintain a healthy blood glucose balance. When you eat, your digestive system breaks the food down into basic elements, turning starches and sugars into glucose. Your pancreas produces insulin, which helps the glucose get into your cells, where it is used as energy. In Type 2 diabetes, the body is unable to use insulin as it should, and your cells become resistant to insulin's message. As a result, glucose cannot enter cells, and it builds up in the bloodstream. The pancreas continues to make insulin, but the cells become even more resistant. Over time, resistance to insulin exhausts the pancreas, which loses its ability to produce insulin. In those with this extreme form of insulin resistance, insulin medication is often required.

Most of the glucose in your body comes from the carbohydrates you eat. Unfortunately, most North Americans consume too many of the bad carbohydrates found in cookies, crackers, biscuits, pasta, breads, and fat-laden foods, and not enough of the good carbohydrates and fiber found in fruits and vegetables.

This high-carbohydrate, high-fat diet is also associated with nutritional deficiencies, (especially chromium and antioxidant nutrients) being overweight, a lack of exercise, and too much stress. Low thyroid function has also been linked to the onset of diabetes. (See Chapter 2 for the glycemic index of common foods.) Always choose foods with a low glycemic index, including fruits, vegetables, lentils, proteins, and good healthy fats. Follow the Body Sense diet recommendations to ensure that you are not overloading your body with excessive bad carbohydrates.

TYPES OF DIABETES

Genetics do play a role in the development of diabetes, but inherited factors alone will not cause the disease. You must also have an environmental trigger, such as a poor diet, too much stress, or lack of exercise, to trigger the genetic traits.

Type 1 Diabetes

Type 1 diabetes, also called juvenile diabetes because its onset is usually during childhood, accounts for 10 percent of all diabetics and affects both sexes equally. In Type 1 diabetes, the pancreas is unable to produce insulin, and in over 85 percent of those cases, the immune system destroys the pancreatic insulin-secreting cells. The pancreas's inability to produce insulin causes glucose to build up in the bloodstream. Because glucose is not transferred to the cells, the cells believe they are starving. As a result, the liver makes more glucose from stores of protein and fat in the body. Muscle is also broken down. Weakness and weight loss occur. The body tries to flush out the excess glucose in the urine. One of the first symptoms of diabetes is frequent urination and extreme thirst.

Type 2 Diabetes

Type 2 diabetes, commonly known as adult-onset diabetes, affects ninety percent of diagnosed diabetics. Type 2 diabetics tend to be over forty, and overweight, although today we are seeing Type 2 diabetes affecting more young people due to the increase in overweight kids. Children as young as four have been diagnosed with Type 2 diabetes. So serious is the obesity problem in our youth that up to forty-five percent of new cases of diabetes in children are Type 2. In Type 2 diabetes, although the pancreas may produce low or normal amounts of insulin, the peripheral organs and tissues have become resistant to insulin's effects. In those with more severe Type 2 diabetes, insulin may be prescribed.

Gestational Diabetes

Gestational diabetes occurs in about two to five percent of pregnant women. Women who develop gestational diabetes are at risk for diabetes later in life, as are their offspring.

Syndrome X

Syndrome X is a disorder associated with abnormal blood glucose and insulin levels along with high triglycerides and cholesterol. Other symptoms—such as recurring kidney stone formation, women with excess body hair and/or polycystic ovarian disease, menstrual abnormalities, infertility, adult acne, abdominal obesity or a high waist-to-hip ratio, elevated blood pressure, high iron levels, earlobe creases, low free testosterone, and low magnesium levels—are also often found in those with syndrome X. The difference between syndrome X and Type 2 diabetes is that although both are associated with insulin resistance, not everyone with the symptoms of syndrome X will go on to develop full-blown diabetes. However, syndrome X is a risk factor for future development of Type 2 diabetes. For more information on syndrome X, read Chapter 4.

SYMPTOMS OF DIABETES

The telltale signs of diabetes are a constant, excessive hunger and thirst, a frequent need to urinate, and weight loss. You may experience profound fatigue, light-headedness, depression, irritability, numbness or tingling in your toes, recurring bladder or vaginal yeast infections, skin tags (see below), and gum disease. Your skin may itch excessively, and your vision may be blurred. People with Type 1 diabetes can develop a serious side effect of the disease called ketoacidosis, which makes them thin (read about Ketosis in Chapter 2). Type 2 diabetics rarely develop this disorder and are often overweight. Symptoms of Type 2 diabetes appear gradually over years. So insidious are these symptoms that most people do not notice them. About one-third of North Americans have diabetes and are unaware of it until they are treated for heart attack, high blood pressure, kidney disease, or other associated conditions.

Another telltale sign of diabetes is skin tags, tiny skin protrusions, which often grow on the neck and face, in the armpits and groin, and under the breasts. Researchers have found that more than sixty percent of people with skin tags also have diabetes. If you have them ask your doctor for a blood sugar test—you may have diabetes.

RISK FACTORS

- Family history, especially a mother with diabetes
- Being overweight
- A waist-to-hip ratio of more than 1 for men and 0.8 for women (see Chapter 1)
- Lack of exercise
- Over age 40
- High blood pressure
- Consumption of junk foods or refined carbohydrates
- Consumption of too few vegetables and not enough protein

INSULIN AND FAT CELLS

Fat cells play an enormous role in the regulation of glucose and insulin. When your fat cells become too large, they send out a number of messengers, like leptin and resistin, that reduce insulin or inhibit its effect (See Chapter 5 for more information on gut hormones.) and also promote glucose production in the liver. Forthermore, overloaded fat cells reduce the secretion of adiponectin, which makes cells more sensitive to insulin, lowers triglycerides (normally high in diabetics), and reduces hardening of the arteries. Throughout this book, my goal has been to emphasize the importance of reducing the size of fat cells that we have packed on over the years. Now that scientists know that fat cells produce hormones and regulate other body actions, they are considered part of the body's endocrine system.

LOW BLOOD GLUCOSE

People with low blood glucose levels (called hypoglycemia) are at risk of cardiovascular side effects, dizziness, blurred vision, and abnormal brain function. Hypoglycemics also suffer feelings of panic, anxiety, and extreme exhaustion. Eating too many high-glycemic index foods causes blood sugar to increase rapidly, then fall just as fast (called the hyper-hypoglycemic reaction).

The adrenals also contribute to the hyper-hypoglycemic reaction. Chronic stress causes the secretion of adrenaline and cortisol (the stress hormone). Both hormones promote a rapid rise in blood sugar, followed by a rapid decline. By following the nutritional recommendations in Chapter 2, including eating small meals that contain predominantly protein and healthy carbohydrates throughout the day, both hyper- and hypoglycemia can be controlled.

DIABETES: DANGEROUS COMPLICATIONS

Complications that arise for both types of diabetes are a result of long-term elevations of either glucose or insulin. If blood glucose levels and blood insulin levels are allowed to vary outside of normal levels for extended periods of time, inflammation results and complications—including nerve damage (neuropathy), blindness (retinopathy), kidney disease, heart disease, and circulatory problems—occur. Over 75 percent of adults with diabetes have high blood pressure. One-third of diabetics have severe periodontal disease. Over 40 percent of new kidney dialysis patients have diabetes. Depression is another side effect of diabetes due to hormone irregularities and brain chemistry imbalances. Natural medicines can play a role in reducing or eliminating these complications.

Regulating blood glucose levels, keeping within a healthy weight range, and consuming a healthy diet can help prevent or delay their onset. However, approximately 40 percent of diabetics will go on to develop related complications. The three main categories of complications are:

- Small blood vessel damage, which can lead to the impairment or loss of vision; kidney disease and failure; and nerve damage, which can lead to numbness and pain in the hands, feet, or legs. Diabetes is the leading cause of adult blindness, and accounts for twenty-eight percent of new cases of serious kidney disease.
- Large blood vessel damage, which can lead to heart problems and hypertension. People with diabetes are four times more likely to have heart disease.
- Infections of the mouth, gums, and urinary tract; other complications including impotence; and problem pregnancies.

All diabetes-related complications are serious. Forty to fifty percent of diabetics will have to cope with nerve damage (neuropathy). Nerve damage is caused by a prolonged imbalance in blood glucose levels, and results in numbness and pain in the extremities. Neuropathy can also affect internal organs, such as the digestive tract, heart, and sexual organs; symptoms are diarrhea, constipation, indigestion, dizziness, and bladder infections. Nerve damage can also lead to impotence, which afflicts about nine percent of all diabetic men.

In severe cases, nerve damage may lead to lower limb amputations. It is the leading cause of all non-accident-related amputations. Each year, more than 56,000 amputations are performed upon people with diabetes. Lower extremity amputation is eleven times more frequent for people with diabetes than for others. There is no pharmaceutical drug treatment for diabetic neuropathy, only natural remedies.

To prevent the onset of neuropathy, monitor your blood sugar and try to control blood sugar levels. In practice it is difficult for diabetics to do this. Even the most conscientious diabetics can experience considerable fluctuations of blood sugar levels once the cells become resistant to insulin.

BLOOD GLUCOSE MONITORING

According to the American Diabetes Association, the diagnostic standards for diabetes are:

- a fasting plasma glucose level equal to or greater than 126 mg/dL
- a plasma glucose higher than 200 mg/d after ingesting 75 g glucose
- sugar in the urine when blood glucose levels are around 160–180 per 100 mL blood

There are two tests to determine if you have pre-diabetes or syndrome X: the fasting plasma glucose test (FPG) and the oral glucose-tolerance test (OGTT). If your blood glucose level is abnormal after the FPG, you have impaired fasting glucose (IFG); if your blood glucose level is abnormal after the OGTT, you have impaired glucose tolerance (IGT).

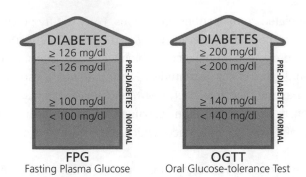

(*Source*: The American Diabetes Association Web site at www.diabetes.org)

INFLAMMATION, FAT CELLS, AND DIABETES

A protein that has been getting plenty of attention lately is C-reactive protein (CRP). CRP is an acute-phase protein found in increased amounts in the blood when inflammation occurs in the body—it can rise a thousand-fold during the inflammatory process. Inflammation is the body's reaction to trauma (cut, injury), infection (from a virus, bacteria, or parasite), a foreign substance (allergens), or damage to the arteries. When inflammation occurs, you may experience pain, heat, redness, swelling, and loss of function—all mechanisms that stop you from using the injured area or alert you of a problem. Combined with other diagnostics, elevated CRP is a risk factor in heart disease (atherosclerosis) and diabetes. Women should pay close attention to their CRP levels; women with the highest CRP levels are fifteen times more likely to develop Type 2 diabetes.

Researchers looking at abdominal obesity have found that as body fat increases, so do CRP levels. Abdominal fat, in particular, is a source of inflammatory proteins—and you don't have to be obese. If you have abdominal fat, your body will produce inflammatory proteins; losing abdominal fat lowers CRP. Certain nutritional supplements—including fish oils, vitamins C and E, magnesium, and herbs such as curcumin and boswellia—also lower CRP.

HELP FOR DIABETES

The following recommendations are designed to improve insulin sensitivity, to ensure weight loss, and to prevent the secondary complications of diabetes. To achieve success, follow the exercise and diet recommendations in this book. Ensure your plate is full of good carbohydrates, essential fatty acids, clean protein (from organic, free-range sources), and adequate fiber. Add an excellent multivitamin with mineral supplement to the specific nutrient recommendations for diabetes. Research published in the *Journal of Epidemiology* in 2002 found that taking a vitamin and mineral supplement reduced the risk of developing diabetes by thirty percent in men and sixteen percent in women. Basic nutrients are the foundation on which you will build your own personalized program to avoid diabetes.

• Eat small, frequent meals made up of predominantly protein? Dietary changes are an absolute priority for diabetics. Adopt the simple rule of not eating any white foods, white sugar, white flour, white pasta, white rice, white potatoes, etc. Eat brightly colored fruits and vegetables because they are high in vitamins and minerals and low on the glycemic index. Regular consumption of fruits and vegetables reduces the risk of developing diabetes. The *Finnish Diabetes Prevention Study* found that lifestyle modification using diet and exercise reduced the incidence of diabetes in high-risk men and women by almost 60 percent.

• Avoid all processed foods. Processed foods (containing sugars and trans-fatty acids) and refined carbohydrates take only a few minutes to cause a rapid increase in blood sugar and corresponding release of insulin. A complex or non-refined carbohydrate can take hours to convert to glucose. That is why we recommend only good carbohydrates. Research published in the *American Journal of Clinical Nutrition* states that women eating a diet high in processed foods containing trans-fatty acids have an increased risk of developing diabetes.

• In addition to avoiding the white foods, attention should be paid to the level of dietary fiber in the diet. Up to 40 g of fiber should be eaten daily by diabetics.

• To increase your intake of essential fatty acids, add regular servings of fish to your diet such as salmon, herring, or mackerel. Eat only good fats and eliminate trans-fatty acids in processed foods from your diet. When diabetics replace saturated fats (the bad ones) with essential fats—from flax, fish, borage, evening primrose, olive oil, avocados, nuts, and seeds—insulin levels are normalized or lowered.

• Eliminate artificial sweeteners (aspartame, Sweet'N Low, sucralose; see Chapter 2 for the dangers of artificial sweeteners) and use stevia (which contains no sugars and has zero calories). Stevia has been shown to have a positive effect on the pancreas in diabetics. Xylitol, which has been researched to prevent periodontal disease common in diabetics, is another sweetening option for diabetics.

• Avoid alcohol and cigarettes. Alcohol is high in sugars. Cigarette smoking increases insulin resistance and high blood insulin levels.

• Eat small amounts of protein throughout the day. When eaten in small amounts, protein inhibits the rise of glucose and stimulates the release of stored carbohydrates in the liver. However, excessive protein consumption at a meal has been shown to increase insulin, especially when consumed with bad carbohydrates. When refined carbohydrates are combined with too much protein—for example, the burger with the white bun—insulin increases. Consume good proteins with excellent carbohydrates low on the glycemic index and good fats, and avoid sugars.

• Avoid or greatly reduce processed meats such as hot dogs and bologna. Aside from increasing your risk of cancer, research has shown that eating processed meats five or more times per week is a risk factor for developing diabetes due to the high content of bad fats, hormones, carbohydrate fillers (wheat, etc.), and preservatives.

• Walking as little as thirty minutes per day can dramatically reduce the side effects associated with diabetes while aiding the return of normal blood glucose and insulin regulation. Losing as little as 2–14 percent of excess body fat in diabetics has been shown to reduce triglycerides, high cholesterol, normalize fasting blood glucose, and plasma insulin. Follow the Body Sense fitness program in Chapter 7 for maximum reduction of diabetic complications. Within six weeks, this program will dramatically change your life.

THE NEW DIABETIC DIET

The diabetic diet recommended by most physicians and diabetes associations is very high in carbohydrates, particularly starches, which are converted to sugars in the body. A better diabetic diet would derive twenty percent of calories from protein, forty-five percent from good low-glycemic carbohydrates, and thirty-five percent from healthy fats.

Michael Lyon, M.D., and Michael Murray, N.D., have written a comprehensive book on diabetes called *How to Prevent and Treat Diabetes with Natural Medicine* (Riverhead Books). They have designed a food pyramid that helps balance blood sugar and insulin:

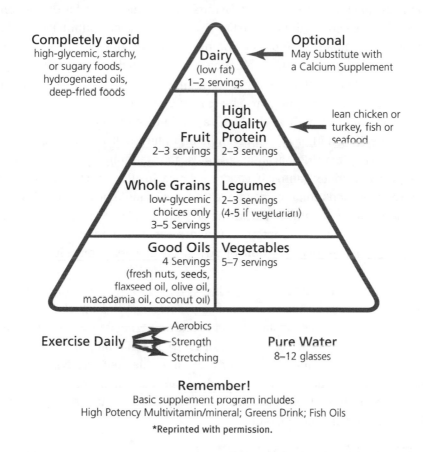

Completely avoid
high-glycemic, starchy, or sugary foods, hydrogenated oils, deep-fried foods

Dairy (low fat) 1–2 servings

Optional
May Substitute with a Calcium Supplement

High Quality Protein 2–3 servings

lean chicken or turkey, fish or seafood

Fruit 2–3 servings

Whole Grains low-glycemic choices only 3–5 Servings

Legumes 2–3 servings (4-5 if vegetarian)

Good Oils 4 Servings (fresh nuts, seeds, flaxseed oil, olive oil, macadamia oil, coconut oil)

Vegetables 5–7 servings

Exercise Daily — Aerobics, Strength, Stretching

Pure Water 8–12 glasses

Remember!
Basic supplement program includes
High Potency Multivitamin/mineral; Greens Drink; Fish Oils
*Reprinted with permission.

SODA POP DRINKERS BEWARE

According to several studies published in the *American Journal of Clinical Nutrition*, the consumption of high-fructose corn syrup is a major cause of obesity and metabolic disorders, including insulin-resistance syndrome. Consumption of high-fructose corn syrup increased more than 1,000 percent between 1970 and 1990, far more than the consumption of any other food. High-fructose corn syrup represents more than 40 percent of caloric sweeteners in foods and beverages and is the sole caloric sweetener used in soft drinks in North America today. The increase in consumption of fructose mirrors the rapid increase in obesity. One reason may be that fructose is digested, absorbed, and metabolized differently than glucose. When the liver metabolizes fructose, it favours the production of fat or the conversion of a carbohydrate to a fat. Fructose does not stimulate insulin secretion or enhance the production of leptin. Because insulin and leptin act as key signals in the regulation of food intake and weight gain, researchers believe that dietary fructose may contribute to the increased calorie intake and weight gain. The reason being that neither of these signals is alerting the body to the high caloric intake of fructose.

Best-selling author John Morgenthaler, in his book *The Low-Carb Anti-aging Diet* (Smart Publications), notes that although fructose has a low-glycemic index rating, it can still cause insulin resistance, increase triglycerides, and promote fat storage. Fructose should be avoided. A study whose results were published in the *Journal of Nutrition* in 1998 found that the long-term consumption of fructose can also promote aging effects including increased production of advanced glycosylation end products (AGES).

An increased production of AGES comes with age, leading to cross-linking of collagen. The cross-linking promotes stiffening of connective tissue, which reduces flexibility, and it allows permeability of tissues and cells. One of the most visible signs of AGES is wrinkling of the skin and the formation of cellulite. AGES form at an accelerated rate when we are exposed to too much sunlight and when blood sugar is chronically high. People with Type 2 diabetes produce more AGES than healthy people; therefore they age more rapidly.

KETOSIS AND DIABETES

In Chapter 2, I discuss the process of ketosis to burn more fat. Ketones, a group of acidic substances, are produced when your body uses fat as its main source of energy. Low- or no-carbohydrate diets promote a natural state of ketosis. In a healthy individual, ketosis provides quick fat loss and poses little concern, but for diabetics the situation is a bit different.

Ketones will appear in the urine of diabetics when they have a severe deficiency of insulin. If an insulin-dependent diabetic is ill or forgets to take insulin ketones will appear in their urine. If the level of ketones in the urine becomes too high, blood glucose levels will rise to dangerous amounts and cause diabetic ketoacidosis, a medical emergency. Diabetics should not follow a very low- or no-carbohydrate diet that includes large amounts of animal proteins. Healthy carbohydrates, good fats, good sources of protein, and fiber are the keys to balancing blood sugar and insulin.

NUTRIENTS FOR DIABETES

The first line of defence against diabetes is diet, exercise, and stress reduction. The following nutrients are adjuncts to a healthy lifestyle. If you are taking insulin, many of the herbs and nutrients mentioned below will lower your insulin requirements, so you will have to keep a close watch on blood sugar levels. The following nutrient recommendations are not in order of importance.

Essential Fats for Diabetics

Part of the strategy to reduce the effects of diabetes is including essential fats in your nutritional plan.

GLA-Rich Omega-6 Treats Neuropathy

Omega-6 essential fatty acids rich in gamma linolenic acid (GLA) including evening primrose oil, borage oil, and black currant oil have been successful in moderating complications of diabetes, including neuropathy.

Not all omega-6 oils contain beneficial GLA, but a healthy body can convert the omega-6 linoleic acid into GLA, and then use the GLA to build nerve structure. Diabetics often have an impairment in the pathway that converts linoleic acid to GLA. The result is a lower level of GLA and its by-products, the healthy hormones. The key to improving the effects of diabetes and neuropathy is to restore GLA to normal levels through dietary supplementation.

Human clinical studies have concluded that GLA has a beneficial effect on the course of diabetic neuropathy. Trials began in 1986, when a group of researchers conducted a double-blind, placebo-controlled study with twenty-two patients. The treatment group received 360 mg of GLA per day for six months. Then a number of variables were tested, including peripheral nerve function, nerve conduction speed, and nerve capillary blood flow. All improved in the treatment group and worsened in the control group. Additional research followed, and two subsequent multicenter studies obtained consistently positive results. The first follow-up study included 111 patients in seven centers; the second included 293 patients in ten centers. The patients received 480 mg of GLA daily for one year. The researchers measured sixteen variables, including nerve conduction strength and speed, hot and cold thresholds, sensation, reflexes, and muscle strength. After a year of treatment, all sixteen variables showed favorable improvement in the people who were given GLA.

Laboratory research indicates that improvement may more complete when GLA is used in conjunction with antioxidants. Alpha-lipoic acid is a powerful antioxidant found in potatoes, red meat, and spinach. It plays an important role in the body's ability to burn blood sugar, thus sustaining normal blood sugar levels. An animal study combining GLA with alpha-lipoic acid showed that subjects had great improvements in the motor skills and blood flow deficits associated with neuropathy. The effects of the combination far outweighed the effects of either supplement used separately.

GLA also stimulates thermogenesis, providing additional fat-burning benefits. Clinical research indicates that a dosage of 500 mg of GLA per day is effective for treating diabetic neuropathy. To obtain this level, you would need 4,000 mg of evening primrose oil or 2,000 mg of borage oil daily.

Fabulous Flaxseed

Flaxseed offers a high content of alpha-linolenic acid (ALA) and large quantities of soluble and insoluble fiber, and a protein profile similar to that of soy. Flaxseed is also the richest known source of lignans. Flaxseed contains so many valuable nutritional components, it is often difficult to determine which component is providing the beneficial health effect.

Flaxseed slows absorption of carbohydrates, because of the soluble fiber and other components it contains and because it slows the digestion of starch. Slower carbohydrate absorption reduces blood glucose, insulin, and blood fat levels, and therefore reduces the risk for heart disease (and maybe diabetes). We learned in Chapter 4 in which we discussed PGX's unique fiber properties that enriching foods or supplementing your diet with flaxseed is a useful way to show carbohydrate absorption. There are a few human studies and numerous animal studies that show flaxseed's tremendous potential in the prevention and treatment of diabetes.

Research presented in April 2002 at the American Physiological Society's annual meeting suggests that diets rich in flaxseed help control weight and diabetes. In the study, researchers fed lean and obese rats a diet containing 20 percent casein (isolated whey protein) or a diet containing flaxseed meal for twenty-six weeks. The obese rats exhibited symptoms of Type 2 diabetes before the experiment. The results showed that flaxseed decreased total cholesterol and triglycerides in both lean and obese rats, and in the obese rats it significantly decreased the bad cholesterol and lowered blood sugar levels. The researchers concluded that flaxseed had greater effects on the variables than did whey, and therefore could potentially benefit humans who suffer from excess weight or diabetes. To obtain the other nutritional benefits found in the seed, such as the fibers and lignans, also take 1–2 tbsp. (15–30 mL) milled flaxseed daily. Fiber is an essential component of any diabetes program (see below). For the complete overview of PGX, a highly researched fiber shown to reduce post-prandial blood sugar, see Chapter 4.

Fish Oil and Fats in Blood

In the longest and largest placebo-controlled, double-blind, crossover trial of the effect of omega 3 fatty acids on Type 2 diabetes, patients maintained their usual oral therapy and were also given 6,000 mg of omega-3 fatty acids from fish oil for six months. Fasting blood glucose concentrations increased by 11 percent during the omega-3 fatty acid phase and by 8 percent during the placebo phase, showing a non-significant net increase of 3 percent. However, fasting triacylglycerol (a fatty substance linked to heart disease) decreased by an impressive 43 percent, a highly significant change. Numerous animal studies have shown the positive effects of fish oil supplements in reducing blood pressure and the stickiness of platelets, and in increasing insulin sensitivity.

Omega-3 fatty acids also protect cell membranes and the numbers of insulin receptors and their receptiveness to insulin. Diabetics should eat plenty of omega-3-rich fish (sardines, halibut, mackerel, herring), as well as olives, nuts, and seeds.

Fish Oil and Cholesterol in Diabetics

People with Type 2 diabetes often have high levels of the bad cholesterol (LDL), as well as lower levels of the good cholesterol (HDL). The beneficial effects of fish oil supplements on cholesterol in Type 2 diabetes was suggested when researchers treated patients for twenty-eight days with 1.7 g of EPA (Eicosapentaenoic acid) and 1.15 g of DHA (Docosahexaenoic acid). Results were encouraging: there was a demonstrated strong decrease in triglyceride levels and an increase in the good HDL cholesterol levels.

The findings of a recent clinical trial published in *Diabetes Care* 2002 suggested that diabetics could partially correct their cholesterol abnormalities by adding fish oil to their diet. The study involved forty-two adults with Type 2 diabetes; some were given 4 g of fish oil containing both EPA and DHA, and some were given a placebo of corn oil for eight weeks. Researchers found that those who took the fish oil supplement lowered their triacylglycerol levels and increased their good cholesterol compared to the corn oil group. The ratio of bad cholesterol to good cholesterol fell in those taking fish oil supplements and rose by four percent among those who were given the corn oil.

Fish Oil for Neuropathy

Fish oil may also prevent diabetic neuropathy similar to GLA. Diabetic neuropathy has been associated with a decrease in nerve conduction and damage to the nerve. One study examined the potential role of fish oil on the sciatic nerve of diabetic rats. After eight weeks of fish oil supplementation, nerve conduction was improved, suggesting that fish oil therapy may be effective in preventing diabetic neuropathy.

To prevent diabetes, you need a much higher dose of the individual fatty acids. Clinical research has used daily dosages of pharmaceutical-grade fish oil of 600 mg EPA and 400 mg DHA.

FIBER AND INSULIN

Brad King, author of *Fat Wars*, expounds on the benefits of fiber for fat loss and blood sugar control. Fiber is found in the indigestible portion of plants: the skin, peel, stalk, seeds, hull, and germ. Its main roles are to absorb moisture in your body, to add bulk to the feces, and to act as fuel for the beneficial bacteria that live in your gastrointestinal system. Even though fiber is derived from carbohydrate sources, the human body lacks the digestive enzymes necessary to break it apart and extract its calories, thus making it a true calorie-free food. Fiber from foods is shuttled through your intestines, where it acts as either a sponge or a mop.

There are two classes of fiber, soluble and insoluble. Each offers unique health benefits. Virtually all vegetables, fruits, and grains contain mixtures of the two types, although one type always dominates.

• Soluble fiber—the sponge—is found in oats, barley, peas, legumes, certain fruits, and psyllium (pronounced "sil-e-um"). Soluble fiber forms a gelatinous mixture with liquid in your digestive system. It can absorb some of your body's excess cholesterol. What gives soluble fiber its grand appeal in the battle of the bulge, however, is its ability to slow the release of glucose into the bloodstream after a meal, thereby lowering your overall insulin response and fat-storage mechanisms. Studies also show that soluble fiber reduces the risk of heart disease.

• Insoluble fiber—the mop—is found in leafy vegetables, root vegetables, and whole grains. Insoluble fiber passes through your digestive tract largely intact. It is responsible for supplying the bulk, or roughage, that keeps foods moving through your digestive system unobstructed (and for keeping you regular).

Fiber helps you feel full without adding fat and calories. Studies have shown that 5–30 g per day of either kind of fiber can effectively reduce hunger. A report in the *New England Journal of Medicine* found that diabetics who consumed 25 g of soluble fiber and 25 g of insoluble fiber per day for six weeks had lower blood glucose levels (about 10 percent lower) and less circulating insulin. The American Diabetes Association recommends 20–35 g per day, but up to 50 g would be better for diabetics who want to control blood sugar and insulin.

If, like most North Americans, you don't eat the recommended 30–50 g of fiber each day, then the foods you eat most likely begin to putrefy in your digestive tract, causing gas, bloating, and increased toxins. Without fiber, foods don't pass quickly enough through the intestines and colon. Instead, they create a backlog of chemical waste that can eventually poison you (a process referred to as autointoxication). Adequate amounts of fiber, on the other hand, keep your digestive system healthy and can really enhance your weight loss.

FIBER AND BODY FAT

Fiber exerts a powerful double whammy against body fat. First, fiber helps slow the release of glucose into the bloodstream after a meal, so it can moderate the effects various foods exert on insulin levels. Adding fibrous vegetables to a meal of higher-glycemic carbohydrates, for example, retards the speed at which the sugars from these foods enter your bloodstream. So, if you have pasta, eat a small portion with plenty of vegetables on top. In a sense, fiber turns higher-glycemic foods into lower-glycemic versions of themselves.

Second, insulin needs to bind to special receptors on muscle and fat cells to exert its metabolic actions. Certain soluble fibers, like guar gum and flaxseed, increase insulin-receptor sensitivity. When there are more insulin receptors in the muscle, there are correspondingly fewer in the fat cells, and more sugars are diverted to muscle cells instead of turning into fat in the fat cells.

Guar gum, derived from the seed of the guar bean, is a great source of dietary fiber. It prevents blood sugar increases after you eat sweet foods, it delays the absorption of sugars, and it has a beneficial effect on bowel movement.

Include fiber from organic fruits and vegetables like celery, apples, rhubarb, blueberries, blackberries, and cranberries in your diet. These foods promote healthy weight loss, stimulate digestion, detoxify and cleanse your intestinal tract, and help remove cancer-causing agents from your colon wall. They also help reduce cholesterol.

Inulin (from chicory extract) is a complex carbohydrate related to lettuce and dandelion. Your body metabolizes it in the same way it metabolizes soluble fiber. Inulin increases beneficial bacteria counts and lowers excess blood sugar levels.

Remember to drink more water when you increase fiber. Otherwise your stool will be dry and difficult to pass.

HERBS, VITAMINS AND MINERALS FOR DIABETES

A tremendous amount of clinical research has been completed using herbs and specific vitamins and minerals for the treatment of diabetes. You will be amazed at the profound effect even a few of these nutrients have in reducing or eliminating your need for insulin and reducing and reversing side effects associated with diabetes. Please monitor your blood sugar when using these special diabetic supplements.

Cinnamon

The culinary spice cinnamon prevents insulin resistance in those who consume too much fructose in high-fructose corn syrup. A forty-day randomized, placebo-controlled trial involving sixty people with Type 2 diabetes examined the effects of 1, 3, or 6 g cinnamon taken daily. Results showed that all the patients taking the cinnamon had a significant decrease in fasting blood glucose, total cholesterol, LDL cholesterol, and triglycerides.

Recommended dosage: Add 1/4 tsp. (1–5 mL) cinnamon to your protein shake or other foods daily.

Holy Basil

In a single-blind, randomized, placebo-controlled trial that was performed in Kanpur, India, the leaf extract of holy basil was found to lower blood sugar levels in people with Type 2 diabetes. Researchers explored the effects of holy basil leaves on fasting and post-prandial blood glucose and on serum cholesterol levels. Fasting blood glucose levels fell by 21.0 mg/dl, and post-prandial blood glucose fell by 15.8 mg/dl. Urine glucose also showed similar reductions. Total cholesterol levels also showed a mild reduction. The researchers suggest that holy basil could be used with diet and drug therapy in the treatment of mild to moderate Type 2 diabetes.

Another benefit of holy basil is its ability to help decrease production of cortisol (the stress hormone) to normal levels. Remember when the adrenals become overtaxed this has a negative effect on blood sugar and insulin sensivity. Holy basil also helps regulate blood pressure by reducing the effects of stress.

Recommended dosage: 100–200 mg three times daily. Look for holy basil capsules, standardized to 2 percent ursolic acid.

Bitter Melon Extract

Bitter melon (*Momordica charantia*) looks like a large, irregularly shaped green cucumber. It is a fruit, not a herb. It contains charantin, which has been shown to be more effective than the diabetes drug Tolbutamide™. Bitter melon also contains polypeptide-P, which has effects similar to the effects of insulin. Bitter melon has been used primarily for lowering blood glucose levels in diabetic patients. The active ingredients in the extract appear to have structural similarities to animal insulin. Clinical trials found bitter melon juice, fruit, and powder to moderately lower blood sugar. Although these trials were small and not randomized or double-blind, bitter melon does look promising as a treatment for diabetes. Researchers suggest that it be taken along with other herbs and supplements that lower blood sugar.

Recommended dosage: 100–200 mg three times daily. Look for capsules containing the whole fruit extract.

Gymnema Sylvestre Extract

Gymnema sylvestre, a plant native to India and used in traditional Ayurvedic medicine, contains special plant sugar compounds, referred to as gymnemic acid. *Gymnema* extract seems to improve the action of insulin; it also reduces fasting blood sugar levels and improves overall blood sugar control.

In a study performed in Madras, India, researchers studied twenty-two people with Type 2 diabetes. All were taking conventional oral anti-hyperglycemic medications. Researchers gave them 400 mg per day of *Gymnema sylvestre* extract. Participants showed a significant reduction in blood glucose, and they were able to decrease their drug dosage over the twenty-month study. Five of the twenty-two were able to discontinue their diabetic drugs and maintain healthy blood glucose with *Gymnema* alone, while the others were able to reduce their drug dosages. The researchers suggest that gymnema's action may regenerate or repair the insulin-producing beta cells of the pancreas in Type 2 diabetics.

Another study published in the *Journal of Ethnopharmacology* found that when 400 mg of *Gymnema sylvestre* extract was given to twenty-seven insulin-dependent diabetics, their insulin requirements were reduced, along with their fasting blood glucose and other diabetic markers like glycosylated plasma proteins and hemoglobin. Again, the researchers stated that *Gymnema* extract appears to enhance the body's production of insulin by revitalizing the beta cells in the pancreas.

Recommended dosage: 75–150 mg three times daily. Look for capsules containing a standardized extract of 75 percent gymnemic acids.

Nopal Cactus

Nopal cactus, also called prickly pear, has long been used in traditional medicine to treat diabetes. Nopal is the most commonly used hypoglycemic food among people of Mexican descent. There have been several animal studies and three preliminary human trials of nopal, and although the results have been inconclusive, it was found that nopal did have a beneficial effect on both blood glucose and total cholesterol.

Recommended dosage: 50–100 mg three times daily. Look for supplements that contain nopal along with other supportive diabetic herbs and nutrients.

Fenugreek

Fenugreek, used for centuries in Ayurvedic and Chinese medicine, has recently shown an exciting tendency to normalize blood glucose. It has been studied in many randomized, controlled, double-blind trials, where it has been found to improve fasting blood glucose levels and normalize cholesterol, among other things.

In 2001 researchers studied twenty-five Type 2 diabetics. The subjects were given either 1 g per day of fenugreek seed extract, or a placebo. In those taking fenugreek, fasting blood sugar levels decreased, and there was an improvement in insulin sensitivity. Michael Lyon, M.D., Michael Murray, N.D., and Dr. Tappan Basu, professor of nutrition and agriculture at the University of Alberta, are examining the potential of various extracts and fenugreek-derived products for the treatment of Type 2 diabetes.

Recommended dosage: 1,000 mg of fenugreek extract daily.

Milk Thistle

Milk thistle (known as the liver herb) is important for those with diabetes because the liver interacts with the pancreas to manage glucose and insulin function. Milk thistle contains a potent antioxidant called silymarin, which has been shown to help regenerate and repair liver cells. It has been used to treat cirrhosis, hepatitis, and other liver diseases.

Milk thistle has also been shown to protect the pancreas from toxicity. It improves insulin sensitivity and inhibits glucose-stimulated insulin release while not affecting blood glucose concentration. Sugar in the urine (glucosurina) decreased dramatically with the use of silymarin. One important aspect of milk thistle is that it does not cause sudden drops in blood sugar but works slowly to stabilize it. Diabetics have been able to reduce their insulin requirements dramatically with the addition of milk thistle.

Milk thistle enhances glutathione, a potent antioxidant; helps metabolize lipids in the liver; and supports healthy liver function necessary for hormone function.

Recommended dosage: 600 mg per day, standardized to contain 80 percent silymarin.

Bilberry

Bilberry (*Vaccinium myrtillus*) is a flavonoid-rich herb that improves night vision; prevents circulatory disorders by strengthening capillaries and improving circulation; and treats kidney and urinary tract disorders, diarrhea, gout, and inflammation. Anthocyanidins are the active ingredient in bilberry. In diabetics bilberry has been shown to improve diabetic retinopathy and circulation problems. Bilberry increases intracellular vitamin C and improves the integrity of small blood vessels, stopping broken capillaries and damaged veins.

Recommended dosage: 20–40 mg three times daily. Look for bilberry extract, standardized to 25 percent anthocyanosides. Take bilberry along with a vitamin C supplement.

Chromium

Chromium deficiency is prevalent in North American society due to our excessive consumption of refined sugars. Chromium is extremely important for glucose-tolerance factor (GTF), the compound that maintains insulin stability, stimulates the synthesis of fatty acids and cholesterol, activates digestive enzymes, and protects the RNA and DNA of your cells. Because of its influence on insulin (and its suppression of sugar cravings), chromium is prescribed for diabetes, hypoglycemia, and weight loss. It also lowers triglyceride and blood cholesterol levels, a common problem in diabetics. Deficiency of chromium leads to glucose intolerance and atherosclerosis.

A randomized, placebo-controlled study involving 180 men and women with Type 2 diabetes, performed in 1997 over a period of four months, found that when patients took 100 mcg of chromium, there was an improvement in insulin sensitivity and decreases in fasting blood glucose levels and insulin levels.

Recommended dosage: 100–200 mcg three times daily.

Alpha-lipoic Acid

The principle role of alpha-lipoic acid (also called lipoic acid or thioctic acid) is to convert glucose to energy. More potent than vitamins C and E, it is able to recycle these vitamins in the body, as well. It is soluble in both water and fat, so it protects your cells (both inside and out) against damage from toxins. In animal studies, it was found to increase intracellular glutathione, a potent antioxidant and protector of the cell, by as much as 30 percent.

The German government has approved alpha-lipoic acid for the treatment of diabetic neuropathy. Considering that conventional medicine has no treatment for diabetic neuropathy, lipoic acid is the only answer. One study found that it regenerates nerve tissue. Lipoic acid also improves blood flow to your peripheral nerves. Lipoic acid lowers glucose levels and improves insulin sensitivity. It also improves your body's ability to burn glucose. Lipoic acid also inhibits the ability of viruses to replicate and supports the immune system. Everyone with diabetes or wishing to prevent diabetes should be including lipoic acid in a supplement regime.

Recommended dosage: 100–200 mg three times per day.

Magnesium

Magnesium is responsible for more than 300 reactions in the body, and its role in the prevention and treatment of diabetes is just beginning to be understood. Magnesium reduces blood sugar levels, improves insulin sensitivity, increases the number of insulin receptors on cells, and maintains the function of the beta cells of the pancreas. A deficiency in magnesium interferes with insulin secretion and increases the rate at which diabetic complications proceed. (Drinking coffee can lower your magnesium levels.) Magnesium levels are often very low in diabetics. When magnesium is given to diabetics, their risk of coronary side effects decreases, glucose regulation improves, and the effects of stress are countered.

Recommended dosage: 250 mg twice daily, taken with a good multivitamin with minerals.

Vitamin B3

One of the B-complex family, vitamin B3 (niacin, nicotinic acid, niacinamide) is an important component of enzymes that are involved in more than 200 reactions in your body. Niacin helps lower blood cholesterol levels and triglycerides. It helps the digestive system by maintaining hydrochloric acid in the stomach and bile secretion, and it can stop diarrhea and gingivitis. Niacin is excellent for cardiovascular health. When a daily dose of 2,000 mg of niacin was given to people who had had heart attacks, the recurrence rate was cut by 30 percent. Niacin is part of the production of adrenal and sex hormones, and it helps the nervous system. It also has a role in energy production, antioxidant mechanisms, and detoxification. It is being investigated for possible anti-cancer properties.

When you supplement with niacin, there is a harmless flushing effect of the skin that can take up to half an hour to go away. If you find the skin flushing uncomfortable, you can buy non-flushing niacin (inositol hexanicotinate). Do not use sustained-release or slow-release niacin: studies have shown it to be toxic to the liver.

Niacinamide has shown some effect in reducing the need for insulin in Type 2 diabetics. It also calms the immune system, preventing the destruction of beta cells in the pancreas.

Recommended dosage: 200–500 mg per day of inositol hexanicotinate (non-flushing niacin) or 25–50 mg per day of niacinamide for every 2.2 lb. (1 kg) body weight. Niacinamide does not cause flushing of the skin.

Vitamin C

Vitamin C and glucose are very similar in chemical structure, causing a competition between these two substances. Most animals convert glucose to make vitamin C in the liver; this provides them with a ready supply of vitamin C and ensures that blood glucose levels don't get too out of control. However, humans cannot convert glucose into vitamin C so we must get it from food. This defect can lead to an excess of glucose in the bloodstream, which could lead to diabetes. Both glucose and vitamin C need insulin to gain entry into the cells. Too much glucose can interfere with vitamin C's access to the cells, causing a vitamin deficiency. Increasing the amount of vitamin C in the diet and reducing refined carbohydrates can lower blood glucose levels and normalize insulin action.

Vitamin C also inhibits an accumulation of sorbitol (a caloric sweetener that is also produced by the body). Too much sorbital can contribute to complications of the lens of the eyes, nerve cells, and kidney cells. Vitamin C, along with bilberry extract, can lower sorbitol levels in the eyes and protect against free radical damage, which also contributes to the formation of cataracts.

High cortisol and low DHEA (an immune and anti-aging hormone) accompany many cases of elevated insulin in people with diabetes. Elevated insulin signals the liver to produce inflammatory proteins. By taking vitamin C along with other nutrients, we can counter this effect.

Recommended dosage: 1,000–2,000 mg per day.

Vitamin C to Bowel Tolerance

How much is too much vitamin C? Robert Cathcart, M.D., and the late Linus Pauling, Ph.D., have said that we each have our own personal vitamin C limit, which is determined by stress, nutritional status, and current state of health. To determine your vitamin C requirements, start taking 1 g doses of vitamin C until your bowels become loose. This will be easy if you purchase powdered vitamin C and add 1 tsp. (5 mL) to a glass of water or orange juice every hour until loose stools are obtained. Once you have loose stools, reduce the dosage until your stools are normal. You will have found your personel vitamin C requirement. Depending on your current health and lifestyle choices, this level may fluctuate from day to day or week to week.

Diabetes Nutrient Program

Remember, diet and exercise are the key to reversing diabetes. The following nutrients are to be used in conjunction with the other lifestyle recommendations in this chapter.

A foundation multinutrient formula containing all the vitamins, minerals, and supporting nutrients for optimal health is a necessary base to which you add other nutrients. Make sure your supplement is well rounded and contains vitamin C, magnesium, niacin, and niacinamide.

- *Essential Fatty Acids*: Essential fatty acids from fish, flaxseed, evening primrose, or borage, or a combination; see the individual essential fats mentioned above for dosage
- *Alpha-lipoic Acid*: 100–200 mg three times per day; 600 mg per day is the recognized dose for treating neuropathy
- *Chromium*: 100–200 mcg three times daily
- *Holy Basil*: 100–200 mg three times daily, standardized to 2 percent ursolic acid
- *Bitter Melon*: 100–200 mg three times daily
- *Gymnema sylvestre*: 75–150 mg three times daily, extract standardized to 75 percent gymnemic acids
- *Bilberry Extract*: 20–40 mg three times daily, standardized to 25 percent anthocyanosides. Take bilberry along with a vitamin C supplement; dosages up to 600 mg per day have been used by diabetics with retinopathy
- *Fenugreek Extract*: 1,000 mg daily
- *Nopal Cactus*: 50–100 mg three times daily
- *Milk Thistle*: 600 mg per day, standardized to contain 80 percent silymarin

CONCLUSION

There can be no doubt that diabetes is a serious disease, but by getting regular exercise, adopting good eating habits, and using supplements, many diabetics may be able to lessen the effects of their condition.

Recommended Products and Resources

In the listings below you'll find recommendations for products and companies that will be able to help you on your weight loss journey.

For more information about *The Body Sense Natural Diet* please go to www.bodysensediet.com

MULTIVITAMINS WITH MINERALS

Multivitamins with minerals are the foundation for your weight loss program.

In Canada: Women, take FemmEssentials™. Men, take Forward Plus™, available from Preferred Nutrition Ltd.

In the United States: Women, take MultiEssentials™. Men, take Dr. Michael Murray's MultiStart™ for Men available from Natural Factors Ltd.

PROTEIN POWDERS

Protein powder is an essential part of your weight loss program. Find a brand that tastes delicious, as you will be using this as a snack or meal supplement for a good source of protein. My recommendations are:

In Canada: BodySense™ ProteinEssentials powder, available in three flavors: vanilla, chocolate cream, and tropical dream. Available from Preferred Nutrition Ltd.

In the United States: SlimStyles™ Meal Replacement Drink Mix with PGX™ in vanilla, chocolate, mango, strawberry, and peach flavors. Available from Natural Factors Ltd.

METABOLISM BOOSTER/
FAT, CARB, SUGAR BLOCKERS

People who have been dieting for years often need some help in boosting metabolism or blocking the absorption of some of the fattening foods they eat. The following recommendations are very effective in achieving that goal:

In Canada: The BodySense™ Natural Diet Kit contains Formula I, the Metabolism Booster, and Formula II, the Fat and Carb Blocker. Formula I contains bitter orange extract, yerba maté extract, green tea extract, cayenne pepper, and ginger root.

Formula II contains Phaseolamin 2250, also known as Phase 2, *cassia nomame* extract, and gymnema extract. Available from Preferred Nutrition Ltd.

In the United States: SlimStyles metabolism booster. Available from Natural Factors Ltd.

THYROID SUPPORT

You will not successfully lose weight if you have low thyroid or subclinical low thyroid. I recommend the following to support healthy thyroid function: L-tyrosine, ashwagandha, guggal, pantothenic acid, copper, manganese, potassium iodide.

In Canada: Use ThyroSense™. Available from Preferred Nutrition Ltd.

In the United States: Use ThyroSense™. Available from Natural Factors Ltd.

ADRENAL SUPPORT

Adrenal nutrients help reduce cortisol, the stress hormone that makes your fat cells resistant to fat loss. Use ashwagandha, rhodiola, suma, Siberian ginseng, schizandra berries or take AdrenaSense™. *In Canada* from Preferred Nutrition Ltd. *In the United States* from Natural Factors Ltd.

PGX FOR BLOOD SUGAR BALANCE

PGX is included in several products manufactured by Natural Factors, including the SlimStyles meal replacement, PGX Control tablets, and WellBetX™ diabetes products. *In Canada* from Preferred Nutrition Ltd. in the GlucoSense™ meal replacement.

PROBIOTICS

Recommended to replenish friendly bacteria in the digestive tract to aid digestion, elimination, and fat loss. Use Bifidobacterium BB536. *In Canada* from Preferred Nutrition Ltd. *In the United States* from Natural Factors Ltd. and Jarrow Formulas Ltd.

ESTROGEN BALANCING

Estrogen imbalance makes it very difficult to lose weight. Use EstroSense™ Available from Preferred Nutrition Ltd. in Canada and Natural Factors in the United States. EstroSense also supports proper fat metabolism in the liver and can be used for cellulite reduction.

CELLUSOLVE PLUS

My favourite cellulite cream, CelluSolve™, contains butcher's broom extract, ivy extract, bladderwrack extract, oil of cinnamon, oil of nutmeg, and dipalmitoyl hydroxyproline (a new compound derived from grafting a fatty acid with an amino acid). Available from Life-Flo Health Products, www.life-flo.com

BIOSIL

BioSil™ helps improve the look of skin, hair, and nails. Clinical studies confirm that BioSil offers superior absorption of silicon and increases collagen concentration in the skin. Available from Jarrow Formulas in the United States and Preferred Nutrition Ltd. in Canada.

WEIGH SCALES

Today you can buy a weigh scale that provides your body fat percentage and total body water percentage. Go to www.tanita.com

COMPANY CONTACT INFORMATION

Preferred Nutrition Ltd.

153 Perth Street
Acton, Ontario
Canada L7J 1C9
Phone: 519-853-1118
Toll-free: 888-826-9625
www.pno.com

Natural Factors Nutritional Products Inc.

1111–80th Street SW, Suite 100
Everett, Washington
USA 98203
Phone: 425-513-8800
Toll-free: 800-322-8704
www.naturalfactors.com

Life-Flo Health Care Products Inc.

11202 N. 24th Avenue
Phoenix, Arizona
USA 85029
Phone: 602-995-8715
Toll-free: 888-999-7440
www.life-flo.com

Jarrow Formulas

1824 S. Robertson Blvd.
Los Angeles, California
USA 90035
Phone: 310-204-6936
Toll-free: 800-726-0886
www.jarrow.com

Tanita Corporation of America, Inc.

2625 South Clearbrook Drive
Arlington Heights, Illinois
USA 60005
Phone: 847-640-9241
 Toll-free: 800-826-4828
www.tanitacom

Index

A

Addison's disease, 16
adrenal glands
  Addison's disease, 108
  Cushing's syndrome, 108, 127
  exhausted, 15-16, 19, 106-114, 117, 125, 206
  fatigue, 29, 86-89, 107, 108
  fight-or-flight response, 106
  function, 16
  function tests, 109-110
  health, 106-115
  of menopausal women, 127
  salt cravings, 87, 107, 113
  sex hormones, 16, 99, 106, 108
  stress hormones, 17, 86, 127
  supplements for, 88, 110-112, 250
  thyroid relationship, 114-115
  see also cortisol, stress
aging
  advanced glycosylation end products (AGES), 234
  excessive exercise and, 198-199
  slowing the process, 178-179
  speeding up, 39, 198-199, 234
allergies, 22, 86, 139, 140
  to food, 18, 19, 22, 140
alpha-lactalbumin, 168
amino acids, 47, 121, 131, 162, 165
  tryptophan, 162, 168
  tyrosine, 121-122
anemia, 134, 135
anti-inflammatories, 9, 136, 160, 219
antibacterials, 132, 144, 168
antibiotic use, 9, 135, 136, 139-140, 149, 157
antidepressants, 111, 126, 162
antifungals, 144
antioxidants, 132, 150, 151, 152, 159, 168, 209, 210, 243 244
antivirals, 132, 144, 168
appetite suppressants, 104, 154, 155
arthritis, 112, 160, 180, 200
artificial sweeteners, 9, 27
athletes, 10, 12, 112, 205
autoimmune diseases, 124, 133

B

bacteria
  Bifidobacteria, 145
  and candida yeast, 141-142
  good, 132-133, 135, 139-140, 142, 145, 147
  infections caused by, 6, 136
  Lactobacillus acidophilus, 145
  probiotics, 132-133, 137, 145
  weight gain and, 2
bad breath, 49, 50, 130, 139, 140
basal metabolic rate (BMR), 14-15
basal temperature, 118, 119-120

beans and legumes
  carbohydrates in, 38, 56
  extracts (Phase 2), 33, 54, 162-163
  as fiber sources, 239
  glycemic index, 36
  as protein sources, 59, 124, 166
  recommended, 30, 58
beta-ecdysterone, 112
beverages
  alcoholic, 20, 82-83, 105, 141, 143, 149, 206, 232
  coffee, 32, 55, 87, 159, 199, 246
  morning, 50, 52, 149
  protein shakes, 84, 104, 165-166, 168-169, 196
  soft drinks, 84, 105, 199, 201, 233-234
  see also juices, tea
binge eating, 5, 6, 21, 83
bladder problems, 138, 165, 181, 226, 229
blood filtration, 146
blood pressure
  low, 113, 122
  test for adrenal function, 110
  see also high blood pressure
blood sugar
  adrenal gland purpose, 86
  and alcholic beverages, 82-83
  bad foods, 105
  fasting levels, 162-163, 164, 229, 232, 237, 241, 243
  glucose absorption, 52-53, 86
  glucose function, 102-103
  glucose tolerance test, 52, 110, 229
  good foods, 105
  high, 102-103, 227-228
  hyper-hypoglycemia, 227-228
  hypoglycemia, 50, 102, 165, 167, 170, 227, 228, 245
  low, 102, 167, 170, 227-228
  monitoring, 229-230
  post-meal, 102-103, 104, 162-163
  regulating, 16, 26, 31, 39, 50, 103, 161, 162, 232
  stevia use, 51
  supplements for, 103-104, 111, 112, 162, 241-248
  see also diabetes, insulin
blood vessels, 219, 228
body mass index (BMI), 10-13
body measurements chart, 26
Body Sense Natural Diet Plan, 59-79
bone
  -building, 114, 171, 194, 219
  loss, 108, 135, 171
  osteoporosis, 115, 165, 171, 194, 200
bowel movements
  diarrhea, 130, 133, 139, 141, 145, 229
  fiber for, 38, 136-137, 144, 238-239
  fowl-smelling, 139
  frequency, 20, 130, 136, 142

index

hormones controlling, 131
importance of water, 135, 201
laxatives, 135, 136
PGX (PolyGlycopleX), 137
regular, 142, 144
speeding up, 52, 53, 168
supplements for, 32, 137, 144
transit time, 136
see also constipation
bowels
colon care, 38, 144
irritable, 130, 149
toxicity of, 142, 148
vitamin C tolerance, 247
see also bowel movements, constipation
brain
aspartame and, 51
disorders, 51, 227, 228
fat requirements, 37
fullness signals, 9, 131, 132, 139, 156
hypothalamus gland, 115
improving function, 50, 111, 112
memory loss, 108, 112, 113, 200
tryptophan function, 132
tumors, 51
breads
avoiding, 58, 104, 143, 197
and candida yeast, 140, 141, 143
carbohydrates in, 30, 165, 224
glycemic index, 35, 36
neutralizing starch in, 162
portion sizes, 59

C

caffeine
and adrenal fatigue, 109
avoiding, 212
excessive consumption, 169, 206
reducing intake, 127, 169
for treating cellulite, 212, 218-219
in weight-loss supplements, 159, 160, 161
calcium, 115, 199
calcium D-glucarate, 54, 151
calories
burning, 14, 45, 46, 178, 179-180, 196, 214
consumption and peptides, 132
old weight-loss theories, 14
cancer
breast, 13, 53, 100, 124, 125, 151, 157, 165, 170, 209
cervical, 151, 208
colon, 157
estrogen-dominant, 100-101, 151, 172, 208
fat cells fueling, 100
H. pylori and, 129
increasing risk, 10, 13, 16
prostate, 124, 151, 157
protection against, 49, 50, 169, 209, 210-211
supplements, 111, 112, 151, 157, 159, 168, 172, 173
candida yeast
antibiotic use and, 139-140
caprylic acid, 144
contributing factors, 139, 140
dangers, 141-142

foods, healing, 143
foods to avoid, 143
hormones produced by, 2, 139
infections, 138-139, 140, 226
inhibiting growth of, 132, 168
leaky gut syndrome, 18, 129, 132
in men, 139
nutritional products, 144
overgrowth, 129, 133, 135, 136, 138-145, 146
questionnaire, 140-141
and sugar, 140, 141, 143
symptoms of, 129, 139, 140-141
caprylic acid, 144
capsicum, 161
carbohydrates
blockers, 33, 250
and candida yeast, 139
complex, 38, 231
conversion to fat, 38
cravings, 2, 6, 27, 139, 162
eliminating, 48
as fuel source, 37-38
function, 38
good, 29-30, 39, 224, 231
high-glycemic, 46, 143
hormone triggering, 6
neutralizing, 163
refined, 38, 46, 82, 170
simple, 38
slowing absorption (find more), 236-237
and thermogenesis, 46
cardiovascular system, 179, 180, 196, 227
carotenoids, 150, 152
casein, 166, 237
cellulite, 203-221
-cleaning juice recipe, 212
castor oil packs, 215-216
causes, 20, 204, 206
classification of, 204-205
detoxification baths, 213-214
development of, 205-206
eating right, 212-213
exercise for, 216
football player's legs, 205
formation, 18-19
liposuction, 218
lymphatic massage, 216-217
oils for reducing, 213-214, 215-216
orange-peel skin, 203-205, 218
reducing, 122, 178, 181, 201, 209, 212-221
saunas, 214-215
slimming teas, 220-221
supplements, 219-220, 251
sweating, benefits of, 214
topical treatments, 217-219
chemotherapy, 140
children
adopted, 81-82
diabetes in, 225-226
exercise, lack of, 83
food rewards, 82
home-alone syndrome, 83
metabolic rate of, 82
obesity in, 3, 7-8, 49, 50, 81-83

of overweight parents, 82
protein requirements, 166
reduced mental capacity in, 121
tips for families, 84, 91-92
TV advertising, 83
water requirements, 201
Chinese medicine, 21, 146, 159
cholesterol
    butter and, 45
    coconut oil and, 44
    HDL, 41, 167, 238
    high, 38, 224
    increasing levels, 40, 44, 113, 118, 126
    and ketogenic diets, 49
    LDL, 41, 104, 167, 241
    liver function, 20
    low, 44
    lowering, 50, 104, 145, 167-168, 194, 241, 246
    normal level, 26
coconut
    butter, 31, 41, 44, 88
    milk, 49
    oil, 40, 41, 44, 45, 49, 56, 124, 143
colitis, 200
collagen, 171, 205, 234
condiments, 31, 56
constipation
    alternating with diarrhea, 130, 149
    causes, 116, 134, 135, 138, 141, 229
    eliminating, 138, 145, 200
    and hormone reabsorption, 147
    and liver stress, 20, 136
    problems caused by, 206
    remedies, 38, 39, 50, 137, 144
cortisol
    abdominal fat, 17, 113, 196
    Addison's disease, 108
    and cravings, 113
    Cushing's syndrome, 108, 127
    in diabetics, 247
    function of, 108
    increasing, 87, 104, 106, 113-114
    liver stress, 21
    in men, 108-109
    reducing, 168
    and stress, 2, 16, 17-18, 86, 106, 107-109
    tests for, 109-110
    weight gain cause, 17, 109
    weight-loss resistance, 2, 17, 108, 109, 114
    in women, 108, 109
cortisone drugs, 140
cravings
    carbohydrates, 2, 9
    causes, 2, 6, 129-130
    reducing, 104, 132, 161
    salt, 87, 107, 113
    serotonin and, 2, 6, 9, 83, 88
    sugar, 6, 9, 83, 86, 88, 132, 140, 141, 162, 175
    uncontrollable, 129, 130

D

dairy products
    alternatives, 143
    butter, 40, 41, 45, 143

    and candida yeast, 143
    as desserts, 59
    glycemic index, 36
    lactose, 33, 38
    non-dairy creamers, 9, 197
    organic, 28, 30, 207
    as protein sources, 28, 59, 166
    tyrosine source, 121
    see also protein powders, yogurt
depression
    antidepressants, 111, 126, 162
    causes, 15, 20, 135, 139, 149, 168, 226
    and good fats, 37, 39
    and liver stress, 21
    and low thyroid levels, 15, 126-127
    postpartum, 117
    serotonin function, 165
    and stress, 17
    and Syndrome X, 104
diabetes
    causes, 38-39, 102, 223, 237
    in children, 3, 225-226
    eating right, 167, 230-240
    exercise, 232, 233
    food pyramid, 233
    gestational, 81, 226
    healing the symptoms, 35, 223-224
    increasing risk, 13, 18, 86, 103, 170, 197, 223
    ketoacidosis, 49-50, 234-235
    and liver congestion, 149
    medications, 223-224, 225
    PGX (PolyGlycopleX), 103-104
    post-meal glucose, 102-103, 104
    pre-, 229
    prevalence of, 224
    protein function, 167
    reducing risk, 231
    side effects, 224, 226, 228-229, 232
    stevia use, 51
    supplements for, 112, 152, 157, 159, 161, 230, 235-248
    symptoms, 225, 226-227
    treatment for, 223-248
    Type1, 225
    Type2, 225, 226, 227, 230, 234, 237, 238, 241, 242
    types of, 225-226
    see also insulin
diet plan, 59-79
diets
    carbohydrate-free, 37, 48
    high-carbohydrate, 103, 105, 206
    high-protein, 48
    Inuit, 37
    ketogenic, 49
    low calorie, 167
    low-sodium, 113
    miracle, 5
    North American, 16, 154
    regaining weight, 1, 5, 6, 158, 204, 206
    successful, 6
    yo-yo, 101, 154, 206
digestive aids, 32-33, 52
    enzymes, 32-33, 56, 88, 137-138, 174

index

morning drinks, 50
digestive system
  antacids, 135, 136
  appetite regulators, 131
  bad breath, 130
  bloating, 32, 129, 130, 133, 134, 138, 140, 149, 156, 239
  chewing thoroughly, 56, 88, 135
  diluting digestive enzymes, 56, 201
  distress, 129-131
  fat breakdown, 39-40
  fiber, importance of, 38, 144, 238-239
  flatulence, 130
  gas, 20, 32, 56, 130, 134, 138, 140, 149, 239
  ghrelin, 131, 132
  good bacteria, 132-133, 135, 139-140, 142, 145
  H. pylori and, 129
  heartburn, 20, 130, 133
  hormones, 6, 129, 131-133
  improper digestion, 2, 18, 129, 142, 165
  indigestion, 20, 130, 149, 229
  inflammation of, 133-134
  leaky-gut syndrome (LGS), 18, 129, 133, 134, 135
  magnesium function, 134, 137
  malabsorption syndrome, 133-134, 135
  nausea, 130
  nutrient deficiencies, 133-135
  peptides, 131, 132
  probiotics, 132-133, 137, 145, 251
  problem causes, 135-136
  stomach acid, low, 135, 139
  tract, 6, 9, 18
  transit time of food, 136, 239
  treatments, 142-145
  ulcers, 129, 160, 200
  water retention, 18-19, 113, 122, 129, 130, 133, 136, 140, 156
  see also bowel movements, candida yeast, digestive aids
dihydroepiandrosterone (DHEA), 104, 106
disease(s)
  arthritis, 10
  caused by obesity, 9-10, 13
  healing the symptoms, 35
  hypertension, 13, 111, 161, 200, 228
  increasing risk, 18
  obesity-related, 9-10, 13, 178-179
  reversing, 195-197
  and trans-fatty acids, 41-42
  see also cancer, diabetes, heart
dizziness, 87, 118, 139, 182, 196, 213, 226

E

eggs
  for breakfast, 57
  eating frequency, 56, 143
  free-range, 47, 48, 105, 150
  protein in, 47, 48, 56, 59, 150, 166, 167, 196
  selenium in, 125
  slowing blood sugar rise, 105
  for snacks, 58
  tyrosine in, 121
emotional eating, 81-98
  affirmations to stop, 92-93, 96-97, 200

  eliminating stress, 90
  food as comfort, 82-83
  food rewards, 82
  journal-keeping, 93-96, 97
  making positive changes, 90-98
  mood swings and, 82-83, 86
  as stress fixes, 85-86
  triggers, 86, 96
  visualization to stop, 93
endocrine system, 111, 115, 227
endurance, 47, 111, 197
environmental toxins, 6, 18, 19, 101, 149, 151, 207
enzymes
  amylase, 138
  aromatase, 114
  betaine hydrochloride, 138
  bromelain, 138
  conversion to lipids, 167
  digestive, 32-33, 56, 88, 137-138, 161, 174
  fat-releasing, 164
  in fermented foods, 53, 125, 132-133
  in foods, 138
  function of, 137-138
  hydrochloric acid, 138
  lipase, 138, 163
  protease, 138, 169
  in sauces, 138
  in yogurt, 138
epilepsy, 49, 50
epsom salts baths, 213-214
estrogen, 9, 19-20, 53, 100
  16-alpha-hydroxyestrone, 208
  -dominant cancers, 100-101, 151, 172, 208, 211
  belly fat, 19-20, 114, 125, 149, 151, 173
  blockers (find more in excess), 208
  cancer-causing, 100, 169-170, 172, 208
  contributing to weight gain, 99, 125
  deficiency and cellulite, 207
  environmental, 101, 151, 207, 211
  excess, 19-20, 53, 126, 147-148, 207, 209
  from candida yeast, 139
  hormone replacement therapy, 2, 9, 125, 126, 128
  imbalance, 101, 117, 119, 148, 172, 206-207, 251
  in men, 19, 108
  mimickers, 207
  in obese women, 100-101
  production of, 106, 114, 208
  reabsorption, 148
  receptors, 169, 170
  in soy, 170
  steroidal, 171
  and thyroid function, 126
  xeno-, 19, 101, 151, 207
  see also menopause
exercise
  abdomen, 184, 186, 190, 194
  activities, 179-180, 189, 195, 196, 216
  for adrenal function, 87
  aerobic, 182, 197-198, 233
  arms, 180-181, 183-184, 186, 188, 189-190, 191, 192
  back, 188, 191, 192
  bodybuilders, 195, 198
  butt, 185, 187, 190, 193

calories burned, 179-180
categories, 47
and cellulite, 205-206
cellulite-reducing, 181, 185, 216
chest and breast, 186, 189
children, lack of, 83
CLA effects, 158
effortless, 180-181
endurance, 47
excessive, 198-199, 204, 205-206, 216
family-oriented, 182, 194
fitness trainers, 197-198
forty-two-day program, 183-194
heart rate maximum, 195-196
immune system enhancement, 198-199
improvements made, 178, 179
injury prevention, 180, 196
intensity, 195-196
and ketosis, 195
lack of, 16, 19, 83, 103, 105, 135, 178, 204
legs, 185, 190, 191, 192, 193, 205-206
light, 47, 87, 179, 180, 198
marathon runners, 198-199
for men, 180
moderate, 180, 198
rebounding, 137, 181, 216
recovery time, 195
right time to, 181-182, 199
running, 180, 195
sedentary lifestyle, 47, 177
shoulders, 188, 189, 192
strength, 47
strenuous, 158, 167
teenage, 47
ten-minute workouts, 179-194, 195, 196, 200
walking, 87, 137, 180, 181, 194, 195, 198, 232
water, importance of, 182
weight training, 197-198
weight-bearing, 179, 180-182, 183-186, 188, 189-190, 191-192, 216
for women, 180
eyes
    blindness, 224, 228
    fatty deposits in, 20, 149
    problems, 21, 141, 227, 247

F
fast, 132
fast foods, 42-43, 58, 83, 132
fat (body)
    -blocking supplements, 33
    abdominal, 6, 17, 20, 87, 103, 104, 109, 113, 174, 230
    athletes,' 10, 12
    brown, 45-46, 99, 154, 155
    determining, 10-13
    factors contributing to, 8-9, 14-22
    factors that increase, 14-22
    false, 130
    as fuel source, 37
    function of, 204
    ideal weight, 112
    leakage, 102
    for men, 11

storage, 15, 16-17, 19, 20, 38, 40, 86, 103, 204, 239
    subcutaneous, 204, 206
    white, 45, 99
    for women, 11, 19-20, 99, 100-101, 114, 125
    see also cellulite, fat burning, fat cells
fat burning, 15, 33, 37-38, 40, 45-47, 48-50, 53, 101
    brown adipose tissue (BAT), 155
    conjugated linoleic acid (CLA), 157-158
    for fuel, 115, 126, 174
    hydroxycitric acid (HCA), 164
    omega-3, 154, 156-157
    omega-6, 155-156, 157
    supplements for, 33, 54-55, 154-175
    see also thermogenics
fat cells
    abdominal, 17, 230
    cortisol link, 2, 17
    development during pregnancy, 100
    distorted, 205
    during diets, 101
    fueling cancer, 100
    genetic problems, 21-22
    high-blood pressure and, 100
    hormone production, 2, 6, 15, 100, 208
    insulin link, 227
    in men, 99
    resistant to fat loss, 108, 109
    in women, 99
fatigue, 15, 21, 87, 107, 108, 113
    causes, 117, 126, 226
    chronic (CFS), 108, 174
    supplements for, 111, 112
fats
    artificial, 18, 42
    blockers, 33, 250
    butter, 40, 41, 45, 143
    coconut butter, 31, 41, 44, 49
    as fuel source, 40
    hydrogenated, 41, 42
    margarine, 40, 41, 45
    monounsaturated, 43
    phobia, 39
    polyunsaturated, 43-44
    recommended, 31
    saturated, 39-41, 42, 149, 155, 231
    sugars replacing, 39, 43
    toxic, 39
    trans, 27, 39, 41-43
    unsaturated, 43-44
    see also oils
fatty acids
    alpha-linolenic acid (ALA), 156, 236, 245, 248
    in butter, 45
    cancer-causing, 169
    caprylic acid, 144
    chains, 45
    in coconut oil, 45
    conjugated linoleic acid (CLA), 54, 154, 157-158
    creating omega-9, 44
    deficiency, 154
    in fish, 88, 156, 231, 248
    in flaxseed, 156, 231, 248
    free, 39-40

gamma linolenic acid (GLA), 154, 155-156, 235-236
hydrogenation, 41
linoleic acid, 45, 157
lipoic acid, 245
metabolism of, 150
omega-3, 44, 53, 154, 156-157, 237
omega-6, 44, 155-156, 157, 235-236
omega-9, 44
omission of, 44
rate, 116
and thermogenesis, 46-47
trans-, 27, 124, 155, 231
see also fats, oils
fermented foods
enzymes in, 53, 125, 132-133, 138
juices, 145
kefir, 28, 145
pickles, 53
sauerkraut, 29, 53, 132-133, 138, 145
teas, 160
yogurt (get more), 145
see also fermented soy, protein powders
fermented soy
importance of, 171-172
miso, 125, 132, 138, 145, 172
powder, 28, 53, 125, 132-133, 145, 166, 168-169
protein, 33, 143, 170, 171
as protein source, 166
sauce, 125, 138, 172
tempeh, 125, 145, 172
yogurt, 125
fiber
and bowel function, 38, 136-137, 144, 238-239
fighting fat, 53-54, 239, 240
flaxseed, 53, 236
guar gum, 240
importance of, 38, 238-240
insoluble, 239
PGX (PolyGlycopleX), 103-104, 132, 137, 196, 236, 250
psyllium seed, 144, 239
soluble, 239
sources, 238-239, 240
fish
eating frequency, 56, 59, 143
eating ideas, 57
farm-raised, 167
fatty acids in, 88, 156, 231, 248
oils, 44, 88, 124, 137, 157, 230, 231, 237-238
omega-3 in, 156, 157, 237
as protein sources, 28, 47, 58, 124, 166
recommended types, 28, 58, 125, 231
for thyroid function, 124
wild, 58, 148, 167
flaxseed
alpha-linolenic acid (ALA), 236
butter recipe, 46
diabetes and, 236-237
fiber from, 53, 236-237
ground (powder), 53, 237
lignans, 53, 170, 236
omega-3 in, 156
pudding, 54, 59
spread, coconut-, 44

flaxseed oil
Better Butter recipe, 46
Coconut-Flaxseed Spread recipe, 44
eating frequency, 143
fat-burning, 56
fatty acids in, 88, 124, 156, 231, 248
other uses for, 41, 137
polyunsaturated fats, 43-44
folic acid, 135
food
chemicals in, 6, 18, 19, 207
cravings, 2, 9, 83, 87, 89, 104, 107, 129
fat-free, 39
fearing, 22
frying, 41
glycemic index of, 35-37
processed, 27, 32, 105, 113, 135, 231
refined, 38
shopping tips, 27, 34-35
soups, 30, 58, 138
starchy, 30, 33, 35, 38, 162, 175
trans-fats in, 42
food allergies, 18, 19, 22, 129, 133, 135, 136
and candida yeast, 140
conditions caused by, 206
food sensitivities, 18, 19, 22
free radicals, 41, 45, 152, 168, 205, 210
fructo-oligosaccharides (FOS), 145
fruit(s)
avocados, 231
bitter melon, 242, 248
calcium D-glucarate in, 152
consumption of, 87, 231
cranberries, 50, 53-54, 56, 221
as desserts, 59
dried, 142
fiber from, 239, 240
glycemic index, 36
grapefruit, 196
lemons, 38, 52, 56, 105, 143, 149, 221
recommended, 29
as snacks, 58
tyrosine sources, 121
xylitol in, 52
see also juices

G
gallbladder, 20, 131, 150, 168, 211
genetically modified foods, 172
genetics, 21-22
glands
hypothalamus, 115
pituitary, 114-115, 119, 122
thymus, 51
see also thyroid
glutathione, 168, 174, 210, 211, 244
glycemic index
foods reducing the level, 52
high foods, 46, 240
low foods, 27, 35-37, 59, 87, 225, 231, 234, 240
gout, 179, 200, 244
grain products
bread replacements, 57
cereals, 30, 35, 36, 55, 58, 143, 165

crackers, 30, 104, 143, 224
pasta, 30, 36, 38, 105, 162, 175, 224, 240
wheat germ, 125
whole, 150, 239
see also breads
grains, 35, 36, 166, 239
gum problems, 226, 228

H
hair
improvements, 171, 178, 219
loss, 15, 39, 116, 135, 164
metabolism of, 206
headaches
chemical causes, 51
dehydration, 200
migraine, 101, 118, 139, 200
as symptoms of problems, 15, 21, 118, 139, 140, 149, 213
heart attack, 100, 126, 167, 177, 226
heart disease
angina, 200
bad fats and, 40, 41, 42
causes, 108, 228
coronary artery, 44
increasing risk, 10, 13, 16, 18, 40, 100, 108
insulin and, 170
protein protection, 167, 168
reducing risk, 35, 236
supplements for, 111, 157, 159
heart palpitations, 118, 169
hemorrhoids, 130, 131, 206, 218
herbs and spices
cayenne, 31, 33, 54, 56, 161
cinnamon, 31, 241
fenugreek, 243, 248
holy basil, 241, 248
recommended, 31
rosemary, 54
high blood pressure
causes, 100, 104, 169, 199, 226
reducing, 38, 110, 157
substances to avoid, 169, 219
hip-to-waist ratio, 226, 227
homeostasis, 110
hormone
-production in thyroid, 9
imbalance problems, 2, 101, 112, 117, 119, 148, 172, 175
replacement therapy, 2, 9, 125, 126, 128
hormones
aldosterone, 106
androgens, 108
angiotensinogen, 100
blood-vessel constricting, 100
cholecystokinin (CCK), 131, 168
crashes, 6
disabling, 9
environmental, 6, 101, 151, 207
factors affecting, 2
fat cells producing, 2, 6, 15
free, 116
from candida yeast, 139

function of, 2
ghrelin, 131, 132
growth, 100
gut, 131-133, 227
leptin, 132, 154, 227, 234
liver function, 19
pancreatic, 131
production, 47
progesterone, 108, 114, 173
progestin, 2, 126
prostaglandins, 156
reabsorption, 147
serotonin, 2, 9, 17-18
sex, 16, 99, 106, 108, 127, 246
synthetic, 116, 149
testerone, 99, 173, 226
toxic, 6
weight regulating, 15-17
see also cortisol, estrogen, insulin, thyroid
human papilloma virus (HPV), 208
hypertension, 13, 111, 161, 200, 228

I
immune system
enhancing, 111, 112, 142, 145, 161, 198-199
impaired function of, 41, 108, 113, 142, 165, 198
regulating, 106, 157
infections
bacterial, 6, 136, 230
bladder, 138, 140, 226, 229
gums and mouth, 228
H. pylori, 129, 136
nail, 138
parasitic, 6, 230
recurrent, 15, 107
throat, 138
urinary tract, 139, 145, 228
viral, 6, 230
yeast, 138-139, 140, 226
inflammation, 133-134, 156, 160, 198, 199, 230, 244
insulin
-related diseases, 38-39
action inhibiting, 102
cortisol secretion, 106
fat storage, 16-17
function, 102, 103, 162
and heart disease, 170
improving sensitivity, 178, 241
ketogenic diets and, 49
no carbohydrates and, 48
rate of release, 38-39
reducing, 106, 231
resistance, 16, 86, 101, 103, 104, 105, 175, 223, 224, 233
stabilizing, 167, 174, 247
Syndrome X, 16, 86, 102, 104-105, 178, 226, 229
use of, 223-224, 225
see also diabetes, pancreas
inulin, 145, 240
irritability, 21, 139, 140

J
journal for optimal health, 93-96, 97

index

juices, 38, 48, 50, 52, 53-54, 56-57, 84, 105, 143, 145, 149
    avoiding, 38, 48, 105, 201
    blueberry, 212-213
    cellulite-cleaning recipe, 212
    cranberry, 50, 53-54, 56, 201, 212-213
    fermented, 145
    for flavoring water, 50-51, 53-54, 56-57, 201
    fruit, 38, 84, 105, 143
    grass, 150
    lemon, 38, 50, 52, 56, 57, 143, 149, 201
    lime, 38, 50, 56-57, 201
    in morning drinks, 52, 149
    pomegranate, 50, 212-213
    vegetable, 144

K

kefir, 28, 145
kelp, 87, 125, 169
ketoacidosis, 226
ketosis, 48-50, 59, 104, 195, 234-235
kidneys, 150, 200, 224, 226, 244

L

lactalbumin, 166, 168
lactoferrin, 132, 168
lethargy, 15, 17, 117, 170
lignans, 53, 170, 236
liver
    abdominal fat, 19-20
    bile secretion, 20, 52, 146-147, 150, 211
    cholesterol production, 20
    congestion, 148-149, 206
    decongestion, 52, 149-152
    detoxification process, 18, 19, 136, 141, 146-149
    digestive system link, 129
    disorders, 151, 211
    dysfunction, 9, 18, 19-21, 147-148, 204
    estrogen elimination, 147-148
    fat breakdown, 20
    fat storage, 20
    fatty, 20, 102
    function, 19, 21, 102, 112, 131, 146-149
    glucose production in, 227
    hormone processing, 19, 115-116, 129, 146, 147-148
    pathway, 147
    stress/congestion symptoms, 20-21, 149
    support, 110-111, 112, 149-152, 162, 172-175, 210
    thyroid relationship, 146
    transplant reasons, 102
lymphatic system, 181, 204, 205, 206, 216

M

meals
    breakfast, 48, 55, 57-58, 165, 182, 196
    dessert, 59
    dinner, 58
    lunch, 58
    menu ideas, 60-79
    protein, 167, 231, 232
    replacements, 59
    skipping, 9, 165
    suggestions, 56-59

    timing, 56, 199
    see also snacks
meats
    free-range, 28, 48, 105, 124
    ketosis kick start, 48
    liver, 150
    organic, 207
    pesticides in, 207
    processed, 47, 143, 232
    as protein sources, 28, 166
    red, 40, 45, 48, 59, 121, 124, 125, 166, 174
    seafood, 28, 56, 105
    see also fish, poultry
men
    body fat in, 11, 172, 173, 181
    body mass index, 11, 12, 13
    candida yeast in, 139
    and cellulite, 204, 205
    diabetes risk, 231
    estrogen in, 19, 108
    exercise for, 180
    prostate cancer, 124, 151, 157
    protein requirements, 166
    testerone, 99, 173, 226
Mendosa, David, 35, 52
menopause
    diadzein, 169
    genistein, 169
    peri-, 125-126, 206, 212
    supplements for, 112, 169
    symptoms, 21, 114, 117, 118, 125, 126-127, 169
    weight gain and, 2, 109, 126
    see also estrogen, women
metabolic rate, 14-15, 115, 116, 119, 126, 159, 165
metabolism
    basal metabolic rate (BMR), 14-15
    boosters, 250
    of children, 82
    jump-starting, 48, 153-175
    liver function, 146
    peak, 15
    regulating, 106, 117
    slow, 6, 14-15, 117
    supplements, 33, 54, 153-175
    thyroid function, 2
mood disorders, 21, 83, 86, 139, 149, 170
muscle
    -building, 180-181, 195-197
    breakdown of, 225
    and fat burning, 177, 178
    increasing mass, 106, 112, 177-178
    lean mass, 10, 158, 163
    overworking, 198-199
    pain, 21, 139, 140
    and protein, 171

N

nails, 135, 138, 165, 171, 219, 220
nasal congestion, 141
nervous system, 37, 111, 112, 114, 115, 229
neuropathy, 229, 235-236, 245, 248
neurotransmitters, 17
nutrient deficiencies
    B vitamins, 134

calcium, 135
causing candida yeast, 139
decreasing liver function, 148
essential fatty acid, 154
folic acid, 135
iodine, 115, 118, 121, 146
iron, 121-122, 134
magnesium, 169, 226
protein, 135, 165, 204
selenium, 135
vitamin D, 135
zinc, 135
nuts and seeds
good fats from, 39, 124
oils from, 39, 124, 231, 237
as protein source, 166
recommended types, 28, 58, 121, 143, 150
and thyroid function, 121, 124, 125

O
obesity
abdominal, 226, 230
body mass index, 10, 12
causes, 1-2, 5, 17, 17-18, 38-39
in children, 7-8, 49, 50, 81-82
deaths caused by, 7, 12
defined, 10-13
determining, 10-13
diseases caused, 9-10, 13, 178-179
emotional problems with, 8
genetic predisposition, 21-22, 81
healing the symptoms, 35
hormone replacement therapy and, 2
insulin resistance, 101
and ketogenic diets, 49
lifespan due to, 100
low thyroid function, 15
morbid, 12, 49
types of, 100
in women, 100-101, 158
oils
Better Butter recipe, 46
black current, 43, 44, 235
borage, 40, 43, 44, 46, 88, 137, 155, 231, 235, 236
canola, 43, 124, 155
castor, 137
for cellulite reduction, 213-214
coconut, 40, 41, 44, 45, 49, 56, 124, 143
corn, 43, 155
evening primrose, 40, 44, 46, 54, 88, 137, 155, 231, 235, 236
fish, 44, 88, 124, 137, 157, 230, 231, 237-238
from nuts and seeds, 39, 124, 231, 237
hempseed, 40, 41
hydrogenated, 43
macadamia nut, 41
olive, 31, 41, 43, 56, 124, 143, 231
oregano, 143
palm kernel, 40
peanut, 43
pumpkin seed, 41
recommended, 31
safflower, 40, 43, 155, 157
sesame, 41, 43, 56

soy, 44
sunflower, 40, 41, 44, 155, 157
trans fats in, 41
walnut, 41
see also fats, fatty acids, flaxseed

P
pancreas, 102, 131, 168, 224, 225, 243, 245
peptides, 131, 132, 168, 242
phosphate, 115
polyphenols, 160
poultry
chicken, 48, 57, 58, 59, 124, 166
cooking extra, 57
cooking ideas, 58
eating, frequency of, 56, 143
free-range, 28, 48, 105
as protein source, 28, 47, 48, 56, 59, 124
and thyroid function, 124
turkey, 28
protein
bars, 84
for breakfast, 48, 55, 165
deficiency of, 135, 165, 204, 206
eating frequency, 56, 143, 167, 231, 232
free-range poultry, 47
as fuel source, 37
function of, 37
recommended foods, 28
red, 56
requirements, 166, 167
shakes, 84, 104, 165-166, 168-169, 196, 241
sources, 47
synthesis, 111, 151
vegetarians lacking, 59
whey isolates, 237
see also dairy products, meats, powders, soy
products
protein powders
for breakfast, 57
fermented soy, 28, 33, 53, 125, 132-133, 143, 145, 165, 166, 168-169
frequency of use, 56, 143
importance of, 54-55, 105, 131, 166
lactose reduced, 33
pea, 28, 33
recommended types, 28
rice, 28, 33
as snacks, 58
sources, 33, 249-250
stimulating the full hormone, 131, 132
whey, 28, 33, 131, 132, 143, 165, 168, 170, 171, 237
proteins
and amino acids, 47, 162, 167
biological value of, 166-167
C-reactive (CRP), 230
complete, 47
incomplete, 47

R
recipes
Better Butter, 46
Cellulite-Cleaning Juice, 212

index

Coconut-Flaxseed Spread, 44
Colonic Cocktail, 144
Flax Pudding, 54
rectal itching, 130, 139
respiratory problems, 107, 112, 117, 139, 200

S

salt, 87, 107, 113
serotonin
  -enhancing supplements, 18, 156, 162, 196
  alcoholic beverages, 82-83
  cravings and, 2, 9, 83, 113
  enhancing levels, 91
  function of, 17-18, 87, 88
  low, 17-18, 88, 113
  weight gain cause, 17-18
sexual difficulties, 112, 114, 126, 141, 224, 228
skin
  acne, 130, 140, 226
  collagen, 171, 205, 234
  dry, 15
  fat beneath, 204
  improvement, 178, 179, 201, 251
  itchy (find more), 226
  metabolism of, 206
  problems, 20, 117, 130, 131
  protein deficiency problems, 165
  sagging, 178, 180, 183, 207
  tags, 226
  wound healing, 165
  wrinkles, 165, 171, 234
  see also cellulite
sleep
  burning calories during, 178
  disfunction, 16, 21, 109, 114
  disturbances, 161, 169, 199
  getting enough, 87, 90, 197
  insomnia, 21, 107, 111, 112, 118, 125, 139, 140, 199
  melatonin, 87, 114, 199
  supplements for, 87, 111, 112, 199
  tips for, 199-200
  waking up tired, 87, 107, 199
smoking, 105, 206, 232
snacks, 55, 57, 58, 104, 196
soy products
  bone strength, 171
  and candida yeast, 143
  daidzein, 169
  estrogens in, 170
  genetically modified, 172
  genistein, 169
  and hypothyroidism, 124-125
  isoflavones, 169, 171
  milk, 36, 124, 143
  non-fermented, 171-172
  oil, 44
  phytates, 170
  plant nutrients, 169
  as protein sources (check p 28 too), 166, 167
  Round-Up ready, 172
  tofu, 28, 48, 56, 59, 166
  see also fermented soy
spices, curcumin (turmeric), 54, 151, 173, 210, 230
steroids, 140, 149

sterolins, 169, 170
sterols, 169, 170
stress
  adapting to, 106, 108, 110-111, 114-115
  causes, 86
  causing overeating, 86-89
  eliminating, 90
  hormones, 2, 16, 17-18, 86-88, 106
  magnesium secretion, 86
  making positive changes, 90-98
  supplements for, 110-112, 122
  test, 88-89
  triggers, 86, 96
  see also adrenal glands, cortisol
stroke, 100, 126, 177
sugar
  -high, 88
  blockers, 33, 250
  and candida yeast, 140, 141, 143
  cravings, 6, 9, 83, 86, 88, 132, 140, 141, 162, 175
  hormone secretion, 6
  refined, 38, 82, 149, 170
  see also sweeteners
supplements
  adaptogens, 110-111
  for adrenal function, 88
  appetite-supressing, 104, 154, 155
  ashwagandha, 88, 111-112, 121, 122
  Bifidobacteria, 145
  bilberry, 244, 247, 248
  bitter melon, 242, 248
  boswellia, 230
  buckthorn, 137, 144
  butcher's broom, 219
  calcium, 199
  calcium D-glucarate, 54, 151, 173, 209
  cascara, 137, 144
  for cell turnover, 112
  for cellulite, 219-220
  chromium, 174-175, 244-245, 248
  copper, 34, 123
  cranberry, 54
  curcumin (turmeric), 54, 151, 173, 210, 230
  dandelion root, 150
  docosahexaenoic acid (DHA), 156, 238
  eicosapentaenoic acid (EPA), 156, 238
  ephedra, 159
  fat, carb and sugar blocker, 33, 250
  fat-burning, 33, 54-55, 154-175
  fenugreek, 243
  globe artichoke, 150-151
  gota kola, 218
  grapeseed extract, 144
  guggal, 122
  holy basil, 241, 248
  indole-3-carbinol (I3C), 54, 151, 172-173, 208-209
  l-carnitine, 174, 219
  Lactobacillus acidophilus, 145
  lipoic acid, 152
  magnesium, 134, 137, 162, 164, 199, 230, 245-246
  manganese, 34, 123
  melatonin, 199
  metabolism boosters, 33
  metabolism-raising, 54

milk thistle, 54, 151, 174, 210-211, 243-244, 248
nopal cactus, 243, 248
pantothenic acid, 34, 122
PGX (PolyGlycopleX), 103-104, 132, 137, 196, 236, 250
Phase 2 (Phaseolamin 2250), 33, 54, 162-163
potassium iodide, 121
probiotic, 132-133, 137, 145, 251
rhodiola, 88, 111
rosemary, 54
schizandra berries, 88, 112
selenium, 45, 125, 150
serotonin-enhancing, 18, 156, 162
Siberian ginseng, 88, 111
silicon, 219-220, 251
silymarin, 151, 210, 243-244, 248
sleep, 87, 111, 112, 199
sulforaphane, 54, 211
suma, 88, 112
tyrosine, 121-122
see also fats, oils, thermogenics, vitamins, and specific type
sweeteners
    artificial, 9, 27, 51, 197, 206, 232
    aspartame (Nutrasweet), 51, 197, 232
    fructose, 38, 233-234
    fruit sugar, 38
    lactose (milk sugar), 33, 38
    recommended, 30
    replacing fats, 39
    stevia, 30, 51, 51-52, 232
    sucralose (Splenda), 51, 232
    xylitol, 30, 51, 52, 232
    see also sugar

T
tea
    black, 160
    for digestion, 220, 221
    diuretic, 220-221
    drinking before bed, 199
    garcinia cambogia, 164, 220
    ginger, 52
    green, 33, 54, 55, 160-161, 209-210, 220
    herbal, 32, 52, 87, 197, 201
    laxative, 220
    oolong, 160
    peppermint, 50
    slimming, 220-221
    taheebo, 144
teenagers, 47, 50
thermogenesis, 15, 45-47, 99, 154
thermogenics, 33, 154
    5-hydroxytryptophan (5-HTP), 18, 50, 132, 162, 175, 196
    bitter orange (citrus aurantium), 33, 54, 159, 161
    cassia nomame, 33, 163-164
    cayenne, 33, 54, 161
    conjugated linoleic acid (CLA), 157-158
    garcinia cambogia, 164, 220
    ginger root, 33, 50, 52, 54, 57, 161
    green tea extract, 33, 160-161, 209-210
    gymnema sylvestre, 33, 164, 242-243, 248
    hydroxycitric acid (HCA), 164

omega-3, 156-157
omega-6, 155-156
Phase2, 162-163
synephrine, 159, 160
yerba maté, 33, 159
    see also fat burning
thyroid gland
    adrenal relationship, 114-115
    affecting metabolic rate, 14
    ashwagandha, 121, 122
    basal temperature test, 118, 119-120
    calcitonin, 115
    candida yeast hormones and, 139
    cold hands and feet, 117, 122
    copper, 123
    dessicated hormones, 116
    dietary changes, 124-125
    enlargement (goiter), 115, 118, 146
    exercise for, 124
    guggal, 122
    hormone production, 9, 114-128, 164, 170
    hormone treatment, 123-125
    hyperthyroidism, 164
    hypothyroidism, 15, 116, 117-118, 124, 127, 135, 164
    imbalance, 11
    improving function, 31, 39, 44, 113, 121-123, 155
    iodine and, 115, 118, 121, 164
    liver relationship, 146
    low body temperature, 117
    low function, 15, 19, 34, 112, 113, 114-128, 164
    manganese, 123
    pantothenic acid, 122
    potassium iodide, 121
    removal, 124
    restless leg syndrome, 122
    subclinical low function, 118, 125, 127
    supplements, 34, 111-112, 121-123, 155, 250
    synthetic hormones, 116
    tests, 116, 118-120
    thiocyanates, 124
    thyroid-stimulating hormone (TSH), 115, 116, 117, 118, 119, 122
    thyrotropin-releasing hormone (TRH), 115
    thyroxin (T4), 115-116, 117, 118, 119, 122, 123
    triiodothyronine (T3), 115-116, 117, 118, 119, 122, 123, 126
    tyrosine, 121-122
    weight-loss problems, 2
triglycerides, 104
    forming, 31, 39
    high, 104, 108, 113, 126
    and ketosis, 48
    lowering, 38, 50, 104, 167-168, 175, 209, 232, 241, 245, 246
    medium-chain oils (MCT), 40, 49
tryptophan, 162, 168

U
underwater weighing, 10
uric acid, 50
urinary problems
    frequent urination, 225
    incontinence, 165, 181
    urinary tract infections, 139, 145, 228

index

V

varicose veins, 131, 206, 218
vegetables
    artichokes, 145, 150-151
    carbohydrates in, 38
    carrots, 29, 35, 143, 150
    consumption of, 124, 231
    corn, 29
    cruciferous, 39, 56, 124, 143, 151, 172, 207, 208
    dandelion greens, 150
    dark-green leafy, 39, 56, 59, 143, 151, 239
    fiber from (find more), 239, 240
    fructo-oligosaccharides (FOS), 145
    garlic, 125, 144, 145
    glycemic index, 35, 36, 37, 39
    juice, 144
    making extra, 58
    onions, 125, 145
    potatoes, 29, 35, 143, 175
    raw, 105, 124, 138
    recommended, 29
    salads, 56
    as snacks, 58
    sodium content of, 113
    thiocyanates in, 124
    tomatoes, 36
    xylitol in, 52
vegetarians, 48, 59
vinegars, 52-53, 56, 105, 141, 213
viruses, 149, 151
vitamin A, 45
vitamin A acid (retinol), 218, 219
vitamin B2, 134
vitamin B3 (niacin), 162, 246
vitamin B6, 148
vitamin B12, 134
vitamin C, 32, 230, 244, 245, 246-247, 248
vitamin D, 123, 135
vitamin E, 32, 45, 150, 230, 245
vitamins, B, 32
vitamins and minerals, 32, 34, 55, 123, 138, 150, 154, 249

W

waist circumference, 12, 13-14
waist-to-hip ratio, 12, 13, 14
water
    after sauna, 214
    for bowel function, 135, 201
    children's requirements, 201
    dehydration, 51, 182, 200, 201
    with detoxification baths, 213
    drinking enough, 48, 50-51, 56, 135, 197, 200-201, 233
    eating and drinking, 56, 201
    flavoring, 50-51, 53-54, 56-57, 201
    hot weather consumption, 201
    importance of, 182, 200-201, 240
    sweating, 200
water retention
    caused by salt intake, 206
    cellulite formation, 18
    edema, 133, 200
    hormone-caused, 140, 156
    leaky-gut syndrome, 18, 129, 133-134
    reducing, 122
    water weight gain, 113, 130, 133-134, 136
weight loss
    cortisol management, 17
    disease prevention and, 3
    products, 5, 10
    resistance, 2, 17, 108, 109, 114, 123, 153
    serotonin management, 17-18
    strategies, 195-197
    supplements for, 153-175
    thought-process changes, 92-93
    tips, 55-56
    visualization, 93
women
    basal temperature test, 120
    birth-control pills, 140, 149
    body mass index, 11, 12, 13
    breast cancer, 13, 53, 100, 124, 125, 151, 165, 170, 209, 211
    building muscle, 177-178
    C-reactive protein (CRP) levels, 230
    and cellulite, 203-204, 207
    diabetes risk, 231
    exercise for, 180
    fat cells in, 99, 181
    feminine hygiene products, 207
    gestational diabetes, 81, 226
    heavy periods, 114, 117, 121
    hormonal imbalances, 101, 117, 119, 148, 172, 207, 211
    hysterectomy, 206
    infertility, 114, 117, 140, 226
    iodine deficiency, 121
    iron deficiency, 121-122
    lactating, 166, 167
    miscarriage, 114, 117
    obesity in, 100-101, 172
    PMS, 21, 87, 107, 117, 140, 211
    postpartum depression, 117
    pregnant, 121, 166, 167, 206, 226, 228
    protein requirements, 166, 167
    supplements for, 208-212
    yeast infections, 138-139, 140, 226
    see also bone, estrogen, menopause

Y

yogurt
    eating frequency, 143
    as fermented food, 53, 145
    flavoring, 57, 59, 105
    good bacteria in, 132, 138, 145
    mixed with protein powders, 33, 55, 57, 59
    organic, 30, 207
    as protein source, 57
    recommended, 30
    soy, 125

Z

zinc, 32, 135, 150